Oral Pathology

SECOND EDITION

Oral Pathology

SECOND EDITION

John L. Giunta, D.M.D.

Professor of Oral Pathology
Tufts University School of Dental Medicine
Staff Associate in Oral Pathology
Forsyth School of Dental Hygiene
Boston, Massachusetts
Diplomate, American Board of Oral Pathology

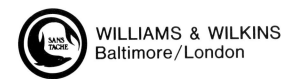

WILLIAMS & WILKINS
Baltimore/London

Editor: Jonathan W. Pine, Jr.
Copy Editor: Caral Shields Nolley
Design: Bert Smith
Production: Carol Eckhart

Made in the United States of America

First edition, 1975
  Reprinted 1981

Library of Congress Cataloging in Publication Data

Main entry under title:

Guinta, John.
  Oral pathology.

  Bibliography: p.
  Includes index.
  1. Teeth—Diseases. 2. Mouth—Diseases. I. Title. [DNLM: 1. Mouth diseases—Pathology. 2. Tooth diseases—Pathology. WU 140 G537q]
RK307.G58 1984   617.6′07   84-2258
ISBN 0-683-03547-9

Composed and printed at the
Waverly Press, Inc.

To my brother,
Paul David,
an astute dental hygienist
and caring soul
and to my cherished wife,
Jocelyn,
and children, Nonna and Weston

Preface

The first edition of *Oral Pathology* was part of a multimodule series of textbooks, *Dental Auxiliary Practice: Biological Basis and Clinical Application.* The original module was written according to the outline and contents of the course on pathology (oral pathology) given at the Forsyth School of Dental Hygiene. Augmented by numerous illustrations, it attempted to give factual, concise information on clinical examination, some principles of pathology, inflammation and healing, developmental entities, microbial diseases, white and pigmented lesions, benign and malignant oral diseases, and some of the oral manifestations of systemic diseases.

This second edition has been updated and corrected in all chapters. (Embarrassing errors in the first edition were noted and corrected.) Several new entities have been included. Intentionally, the common conditions and diseases along with normal findings have been emphasized. Utilizing oral diseases, principles of pathology have been introduced. Purposely this is not a complete text on oral pathology. Numerous excellent textbooks cover the subject in greater depth and emphasis. Consequently, there is limited coverage of areas such as developmental syndromes, bone diseases, and many other systemic diseases. There is no coverage of periodontal disease since it demands a separate course and text. Nonetheless, it is hoped that this textbook will again be servicable as an aid in understanding some basic pathology and oral pathology and as a review for those wanting a short, well illustrated and practical book.

I would like to acknowledge my teachers, Dr. Gerald Shklar and Dr. Edmund Cataldo, for their education and the opportunity to do this work and for some of the photographs; Dr. Esther Wilkins-Gallagher for her encouragement and her persuasion for me to add my own artwork; Dr. Gayanne DeVry for the original artwork; and Mary Hayward for her conscientious secretarial help. In addition, I thank Drs. Kabani and Plourde for the photographs on amelogenesis imperfecta.

Contents

Preface vii

Chapter 1 Clinical Examination   1

Chapter 2 Principles of Pathology   11

Chapter 3 Inflammation and Repair   19

Chapter 4 Developmental Abnormalities   27

Chapter 5 Caries and Dental Pulp Disorders   46

Chapter 6 Oral Mucous Membrane Pathology   70

Chapter 7 Benign and Malignant Conditions 111

Chapter 8 Oral Manifestations of Systemic Diseases 132

Bibliography 137

Index 139

Clinical Examination

The dental auxiliary, as a member of the health team, is responsible for understanding and recognizing diseases of the teeth and adjacent tissues and disorders of the oral cavity and paraoral area. This knowledge is based on principles of pathology as they relate to the head, neck, and oral stuctures.

The auxiliary can readily observe the patient at each appointment. By a carefully planned routine examination, the auxiliary will be able to recognize several disease states. Many conditions can be diagnosed readily when they are first observed; others will present as characteristic lesions that may suggest several disease entities. In these cases further information will be required for a definite diagnosis. The dental auxiliary should note and record the observations and should refer those cases that require further diagnosis and treatment to other members of the oral health team.

Observation is the key in maintaining oral health. The head, neck, and oral cavity are areas that can be easily viewed. Both normal and abnormal states of the soft tissue can be inspected by eye alone. Thus, with an understanding of disease states and changes that can occur, the dental auxiliary can detect disease entities which may be present. It is the purpose of this book to acquaint auxiliary personnel with several aspects of disease states with emphasis on those appearing in the oral regions.

EXAMINATION PROCEDURE

With knowledge of what is normal and of what one expects to see, the auxiliary can routinely perform a systematic examination of the patient. This simple procedure will take no longer than a few minutes and may yield fruitful information regarding the health status of this area of the body. To be effective the examination must be *routine*, *preplanned*, and *orderly*. It should be done at every visit. By using the same sequence of steps at each examination, the examiner will not inadvertently avoid any area. The specific order to be used is a matter of individual choice for each examiner. However, regardless of the order chosen, it is of utmost importance to start in the same site every time and to move in a predetermined pattern.

Utilizing primarily inspection and palpation, the following method of examination is offered as a basis for establishing a logical order and sequence.

Extraoral examination
1. Generalized appraisal of the patient
2. Face
3. Submental and submandibular lymph node areas
4. Parotid glands
5. Temporomandibular joint area
6. Ears
7. Neck and cervical lymph node areas
8. Thyroid gland area

Oral examination
1. Lips and corners of mouth
2. Mucous membrane of lips, labial and buccal vestibulae, gingivae, buccal mucosa, and papillae of parotid ducts
3. Hard palate and palatal gingivae
4. Soft palate

5. Tonsillar areas and posterior pharynx
6. Tongue—dorsum, lateral borders
7. Tongue—ventrum
8. Floor of mouth and lingual gingivae
9. Teeth (occlusion, caries)

The materials required for this examination are a good light, a dental mirror, 2 × 2 gauze, and an explorer. The patient should be asked to remove eyeglasses, earrings, and any other removable items such as dental prostheses.

EXAMINATION TECHNIQUE

The clinical examination of the patient should begin with a general overall evaluation of the individual. The patient should be observed while walking to the dental chair. This may yield information on the attitude of the patient and of obvious physical problems which may be discussed with the patient. This casual examination takes place prior to seating the patient and before obtaining any history. For example, swollen ankles may indicate edema due to a kidney or a heart problem. After reviewing the medical and dental history, the examination should proceed.

On viewing and palpating the face, the examiner should observe if there is normal symmetry. An asymmetry of the face could be due to a swelling related to an abscessed tooth. Excluding trauma, the most common cause of facial swelling is dental in origin. Pigmented lesions such as moles and age spots and ulcers such as skin cancers are readily observable and should be questioned (Figs. 1.1 and 1.2). A rash on the skin of the face may be due to allergy. That a patient has allergies is most important in gathering further historical data that could have a direct bearing on treatment. Some asymmetries can be due to swollen lymph nodes. Whether or not they are swollen, lymph node areas should be palpated.

Lymph nodes are organs of defense that react to inflammation, infection and tumors by enlarging. For example, in an infection such as primary herpetic gingivosto-

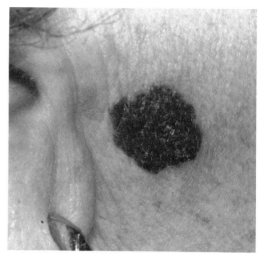

Figure 1.1. Malignant melanoma anterior to right ear. Note dark color and irregular border. Also note paler, even-bordered lesion posterior to melanoma, a common "age-spot".

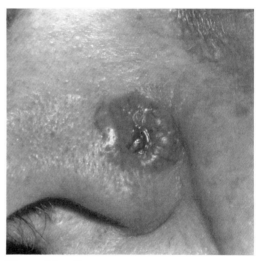

Figure 1.2. Basal cell tumor on left side of nose. A nonhealing crater-like ulcer with shiny, rolled margins.

matitis, several nodes in many sites in the neck will enlarge and be tender. After the disease passes, the nodes gradually regress in size and become asymptomatic. Multiple inflammatory episodes may cause the node to develop sufficient scar tissue or growth so that the node remains enlarged even though there is no stimulus for reaction. Thus the significance of palpating a node (positive lymphadenopathy) may not always be readily apparent until coupled with other physical findings. If palpable, the nodes may be tender or nontender, mobile, or fixed to the adjacent tissues. Malignant tumors can spread to lymph nodes and grow in them, causing permanent enlargement and fixation of the node.

In their normal state, lymph nodes are nontender, soft and cannot be felt unless there is residual enlargement. Therefore, the examiner proceeds to feel beneath the skin for them in their prescribed anatomi-cal areas (Fig. 1.3). Starting from the sub-mental area (Fig. 1.4), one then moves posteriorly to the submandibular area (Figs. 1.5 and 1.6), the parotid region, the ears and then to the neck. Bimanual palpation is recommended, and for the submandibular area this can be done both intra- and extraorally.

The parotid glands can be palpated for swellings. If the patient clenches the teeth together, any swellings of the parotid area can be felt over the firm masseter muscle. Sometimes the masseter muscles are so

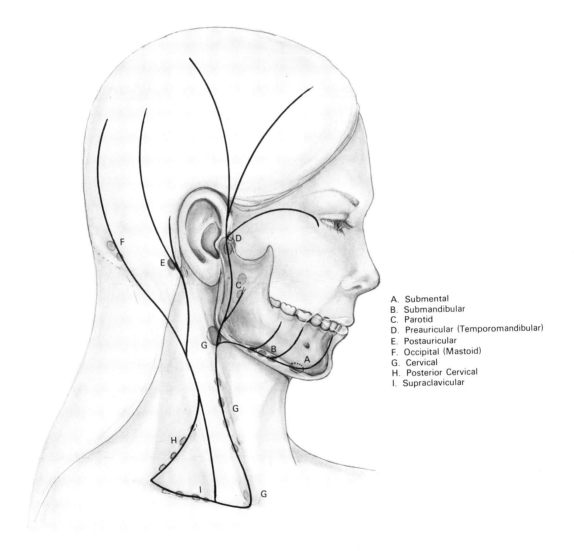

A. Submental
B. Submandibular
C. Parotid
D. Preauricular (Temporomandibular)
E. Postauricular
F. Occipital (Mastoid)
G. Cervical
H. Posterior Cervical
I. Supraclavicular

Figure 1.3. Simplified diagrammatic drawing of lymph glands of the head and neck.

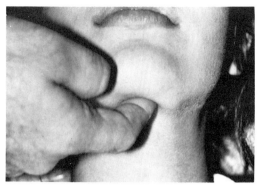

Figure 1.4. Palpation of submental area.

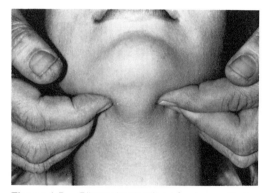

Figure 1.5. Bilateral palpation of submandibular gland area.

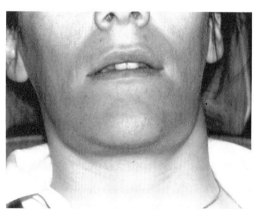

Figure 1.6. Bilateral swellings of reactive submandibular lymph nodes in 24-year-old with primary herpetic gingivostomatitis.

large that they resemble swellings of the parotid area. Next, the temporomandibular joint area can be palpated in front of the ear opening while the patient opens and

closes the jaw. Any cracking or history of pain should be noted. Following this, the area behind the ears should be examined. Not infrequently a tumor or sore may be located there.

Then the cervical and neck nodes should be palpated. By tracing the extent of the sternocleidomastoid muscle both superficially and deeply, these nodes may be felt (Figs. 1.7 and 1.8). Positive posterior auricular and occipital lymphadenopathy combined with swollen, sore palatine tonsils is strongly suggestive of infectious mononucleosis (Fig. 1.9). Positive supraclavicular lymphadenopathy can mean that there is a malignant disease from the mediastinum or from the thyroid gland. The thyroid gland itself and abnormalities can be palpated with the hand over the midline of the neck; when the patient swallows, the gland passes under the hand.

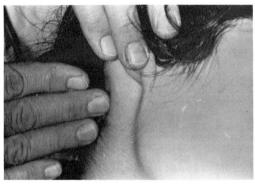

Figure 1.7. Inspection behind ear and palpation of postauricular area.

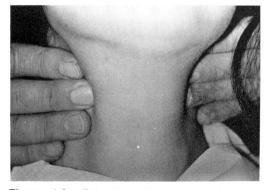

Figure 1.8. Palpation of cervical node area along sternocleidomastoid muscle.

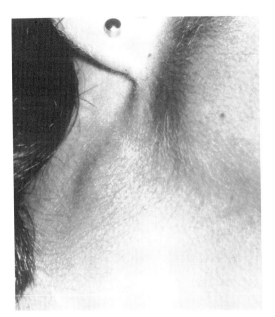

Figure 1.9. Swollen postauricular lymph node in 18-year-old with infectious mononucleosis. The palatine tonsils were also swollen, tender and necrotic.

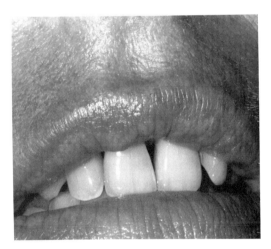

Figure 1.10. Fordyce's glands, ectopic sebaceous glands, on inner aspect of upper lip.

In beginning the oral examination, first note the lips. A scar on the skin surface may represent the closure of a cleft lip or repair from an accident. Frequently yellow glands will show through the vermilion border (Fig. 1.10). Next, after having the patient bring the teeth together (this relaxes the lip muscle), grasp the lips and reflect them to visualize the whole mucosal surface. The maxillary frenum will be a normal landmark at the base of the upper lip. Freqently, there is a small tab of extranormal tissue attached to the frenum (Fig. 1.11). In a similar manner, the lower lip is pulled down and inspected (Fig. 1.12). If this surface is dried, the tiny openings of mucous ducts will be seen and will express drops of mucus. Then proceed first on one side and then the other to view the labial and buccal vestibules along with the unattached and attached gingivae (Fig. 1.13).

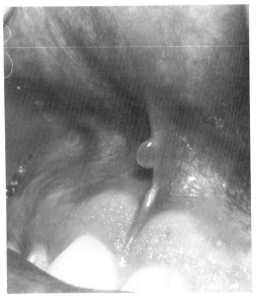

Figure 1.11. A normal mucosal tag projecting from the maxillary labial frenum. Also note normal mucogingival line and stippled gingivae.

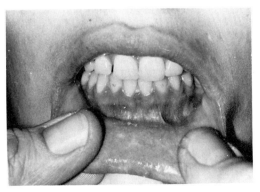

Figure 1.12. Retraction of lower lip.

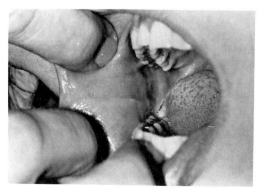

Figure 1.13. Examination of buccal mucosa. Note occlusal or bite line.

Next, reflect the corner of the mouth to expose the buccal mucosa (inner cheeks). Here there are two landmarks. One is the papilla and opening of the parotid (Stensen's) duct of the parotid gland. A clear saliva usually can be seen flowing from the opening (Fig. 1.14). The flow can be tested by squeezing the area of the parotid gland over the posterior lateral border of the ramus of the mandible. The other landmark is not anatomical but is found consistently. This is the white line corresponding to the occlusal or bite line of the teeth and is seen in the middle of the cheek running from the back to the front of the mouth.

Next the hard palate can be viewed, either directly or with the dental mirror (Fig. 1.15). The anterior portion contains the folds of tissue called rugae. Posteriorly, it is whitened due to the keratinized surface. Laterally, where there are numerous minor salivary glands and a prominent vascularity, there is an underlying blueness. The ductal openings are pin-sized and pink. In smokers, they may be reddened and more prominent. A white line can be seen in the midline because there are no glands or fat there, and the connective tissue is bound tightly to the firm bone beneath this area. Frequently, there can be excess bone in this area of the hard palate (torus) (Fig. 1.16).

Moving toward the posterior, the examiner should see the soft palate in its entirety (Fig. 1.17). This includes visualizing the full extent of the pendulous uvula. In this region are many of the oral tonsillar tissues

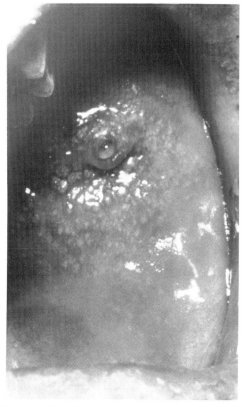

Figure 1.14. A prominent papilla of Stensen's duct with clear, watery saliva coming from the parotid gland. Also note the ectopic sebaceous glands within the buccal mucosa.

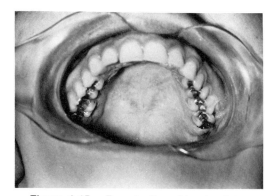

Figure 1.15. Examination of hard palate.

(Fig. 1.18). The most prominent are the palatine tonsils on each side situated between the palatoglossal and the palatopharyngeal folds. They may be very large in children but in adults they should be receded between the folds unless they are

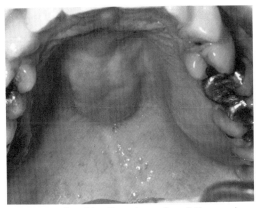

Figure 1.16. Maxillary torus in midline and exostosis on the left lingual alveolar ridge. Both are bony projections and are painless and solid to touch.

enlarged by reactivity or tumor. The tonsillar crypts are indentations that can become filled with bacteria. A bacterial plug is a yellow accumulation of bacteria filling the crypt and may cause a tickle in the throat. Another yellow lesion frequently seen is the pseudocyst. If the epithelium at the opening of the crypt fuses, then the normally desquamating cells lining the crypt pile up and expand forming a cystlike, yellow lesion (Fig. 1.19). Pseudocysts can

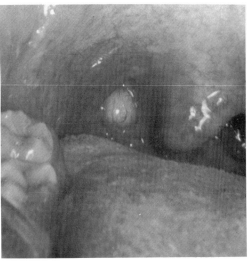

Figure 1.19. Pseudocyst of the right palatine tonsil. Bright yellow, it resembled a fatty tumor, a lipoma.

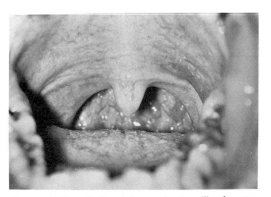

Figure 1.17. Soft palate, uvula, tonsillar fauces, and posterior pharynx, including enlarged pharyngeal tonsils (*at right*).

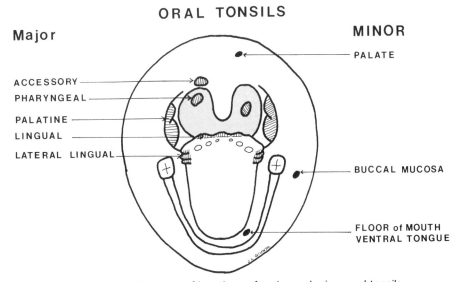

Figure 1.18. Diagram of locations of major and minor oral tonsils.

occur in any oral tonsillar tissue and usually spontaneously regress so they do not have to be removed.

Also seen in this area, but not consistently, are the accessory tonsils. They usually are near the base of the uvula and resemble a tumor such as a fibroma. However, that they decrease in size after being reactive is a clue to their tonsillar nature. If the palatine tonsils have been surgically removed, there may be broad white bands of scar tissue or even fenestrations in the tissue. Not infrequently, there are "residual" nodules of reactive tonsil that remain and enlarge after the palatine tonsils are "removed" (Fig. 1.20)

By reflecting the tongue down and foward with the dental mirror and by asking the patient to say "ah," with good light, the uvular tonsillar area and pharyngeal wall can be noted. Patients with colds may have red streaks in the mucosa in this area.

The tongue should be viewed next (Fig. 1.21). The dorsal surface can be seen easily by asking the patient to extend the tongue. Several aspects of anatomy should be noted. The white "coating," which may be accentuated in some diseases, represents the individual filiform papillae of the tongue. These may be stained brown in heavy smokers or tea drinkers. Interspersed among these are small pink dome-shaped fungiform, papillae (Fig. 1.22). These may be quite prominent in some individuals, particularly in disease states in which the

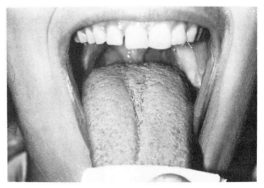

Figure 1.21. Retraction of tongue with gauze. Note filiform papillae (white "hairs").

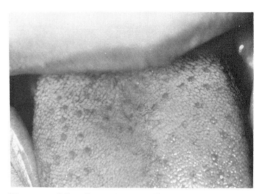

Figure 1.22. Dorsal view of tongue. Note small dome-shaped fungiform papillae among white filiform papillae.

filiform papillae are absent. The circumvallate papillae usually are not seen. When they are seen, they appear as large swellings on the posterior surface of the tongue (Fig. 1.23). Because they occur symmetrically and bilaterally in the form of a "V" with the point toward the pharynx, they can usually be distinguished from a pathologic swelling which is usually unilateral.

The tongue can be viewed easily and controlled well by holding it with 2 × 2 gauze wrapped around the tip of the tongue. In this manner, the examiner can draw the tongue to each side and view the lateral aspects. The lateral lingual tonsil area, just forward of the extreme posterolateral border, should be noted (Figs. 1.24 and 1.25). Bilateral they are nodular with vertical crypts and may be swollen and reddened, particularly in smokers.

The patient should then be asked to touch the palate with the tongue. By doing

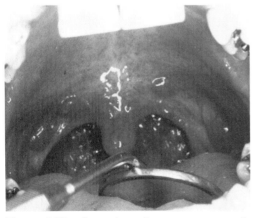

Figure 1.20. Several swollen accessory tonsils on each side of uvula.

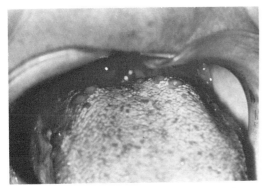

Figure 1.23. Posterior dorsum of tongue. Note large circumvallate papillae.

this, the ventral surface of the tongue and the floor of the mouth can be visualized (Fig. 1.26). Some patients cannot touch the roof of the mouth because of the manner in which the lingual frenum attaches to the tongue (tongue-tie). Not only will the examiner see the lingual frenum, but he will also note the large veins running laterally on each side. These become more prominent in elderly patients. Analogous to varicose veins of the lower legs, they are called lingual varicosities or varices, due to loss of elastic tissue in the vein causing a distention (Fig. 1.27). Then the floor of the mouth

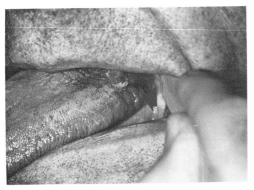

Figure 1.24. Posterior lateral aspect of tongue. Lateral lingual tonsil (foliate papillae) at arrow.

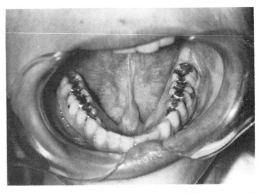

Figure 1.26. Floor of mouth, lingual frenum, and gingivae.

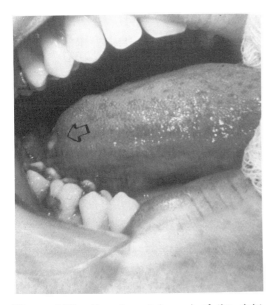

Figure 1.25. Pseudocyst (*arrow*) of the right lateral lingual tonsil. It was yellow, painless, non-removable and regressed in 2 months.

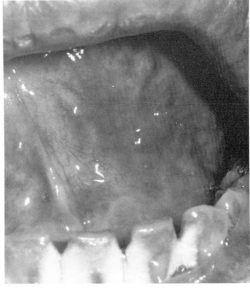

Figure 1.27. Varicosities of veins in ventral surface of tongue. They resemble a tumor of blood vessels, a hemangioma.

is examined. In the anterior portion on each side are the sublingual plicae, or carunculae, which are slightly raised horizontal cylinders of tissue with openings of lingual glands at the surface. Shaped like a "V" pointing toward the anterior teeth, these folds end at a slightly larger swelling with a large ductal opening [submandibular (Wharton's) duct (Fig. 1.28)]. Saliva can be readily expressed from these openings by pressing the submandibular glands against the lower borders of the mandible. Sometimes a stone may form in one of the ducts and the flow will be impeded or stopped. If there is an edentulous alveolar ridge with substantial resorption, the floor of the mouth may resemble a swelling (Fig. 1.29).

With a dental mirror and direct viewings, the unattached and attached gingivae should be noted (Fig. 1.30). Next, the teeth should be checked. After asking the patient to close the teeth together, observe for possible malocclusion. With an explorer, the examiner can check for caries and other defects.

Through routine examination such as

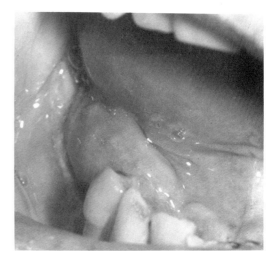

Figure 1.29. Floor of mouth resembling a tumor. The edentulous ridge is so resorbed that normal tissue projects above it.

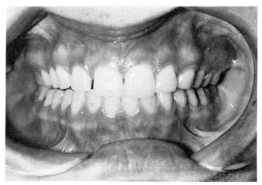

Figure 1.30. Labial and buccal vestibule, gingivae, and teeth.

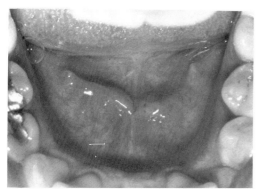

Figure 1.28. Normal floor of mouth showing sublingual carunculae. Note the opening of Wharton's duct near the midline.

this (i.e. methodically and consistently performed), any deviations from normal can be observed. These may range from simple and innocuous defects to very serious and lethal diseases. What is important is that these deviations are observed. The welfare of the patient will be enhanced because of astute observation and referral.

CHAPTER 2

Principles of Pathology

Pathology is the study of the nature of disease, its causes (etiology), development (pathogenesis), and consequences (prognosis). Disease is defined as any abnormal condition of an organism or one of its parts, especially as a consequence of inherent weakness, physical stimuli, infection, emotional stress, or other factor that may impair normal physiologic functioning. Oral pathology is that branch of pathology that deals specifically with diseases affecting the oral areas—the teeth, adjacent tissues, oral mucosa, and contiguous parts. However, the underlying tissue and cellular reactions that produce the morphologic (concerning structure and form) and physiologic (functional) changes in the oral region are the same basic responses that occur in any other area of the body. Therefore a study of oral disease will cover principles of pathology that apply to disease anywhere in the body.

Historically, the nature of disease was a mystery until the advent of the microscope and its application to the study of diseased tissue. Through the microscope it was discovered that organs and tissues are composed of cells and that changes in the cells are responsible for changes in the organs. The altered functional state of cells led to cellular structural changes in many disease states which the early pathologists began to categorize and classify.

Classification of a disease is a valuable means of identifying a particular disease or type of disease. However, it should be remembered that classification is arbitrary. Many diseases can be classified in many

ways. For example, mumps, because it is caused by a virus, can be classed as a viral disease. On the other hand, mumps affect glandular tissue and can be classed as a salivary gland disease. The point is that a classification is a man-made convenience so that disease can be thought of and discussed with some order. The approach in this book will be mainly morphologic with particular emphasis on the gross manifestations of various abnormal states. In some instances reference will be made to microscopic features because certain disease states can be appreciated only in microscopic terms. One should keep in mind that we are in an era of biochemistry and many diseases cannot be recognized simply on a morphologic basis but require sophisticated means to determine their presence, especially the metabolic disease states. With the increase in technologic applications, more and more abnormal conditions will be discovered. Regardless of the approach to the study of disease, certain principles emerge.

Organs and tissues are composed of cells in a fluid environment. Physiologically the cell is a small machine that is capable of specific work but requires nutrients and oxygen to perform its function. The nutrients are derived from the alimentary canal and the oxygen comes from the lungs. The blood vessels carry the nutrients and oxygen to the cells via the surrounding fluid medium. The cell utilizes the nutrients and through metabolism burns the oxygen to produce energy for its work. Waste products including carbon dioxide are excreted by the cell and enter the venous drainage. The carbon dioxide travels to the lungs where it is exchanged for oxygen. The other waste products are broken down in the liver and kidney and are excreted in the urine.

Etiology refers to the cause of disease. There are many etiologic agents that can injure the host and, ultimately, the reaction of the host to the injury produces signs and symptoms of what is recognized as disease. There is a long list of factors that produce injury but the reaction of the host in response to these factors is limited. Usually, many injurious agents act on the host by producing a similar or common response.

The etiologic agents are many but can be essentially categorized as endogenous and exogenous. Endogenous refers to those injuries occurring within the cell. These are primarily genetic and constitute hereditary disease. However, there are spontaneous changes that can take place inside the cell and these changes are not passed on to further generations.

Exogenous refers to those factors originating outside the cell itself. These agents are the most common ones producing disease. They include such stimuli as trauma, drugs, temperature, radiation, parasites (viruses, bacteria, fungi), nutrition, and emotion.

Once one of these agents affects the host, the host's cells are stimulated to react. The response usually takes one of a limited number of patterns that have been categorized utilizing the light microscope. As the cells adjust to the injury, alterations can be seen in the cells. Certain cell types become more prominent than other cell types. Cells may take a specific direction of growth and maturation. With the variation in the external environment, cells adjust and the cellular adjustments assume certain patterns that can be recognized and labeled in a consistent manner. This labeling has led to the categorization of diseases which serves as a useful diagnostic tool. The responses of the host to injurious agents are outlined in Table 2.1.

Malformations occur primarily from agents injuring the inside of the cell and include both hereditary and developmental

Table 2.1.
Pathologic stimulating factors and responses in host

Factors	Possible responses in host (major categories of disease)
Injury	A. *Malformations* Inborn errors (metabolic) hereditary (genetic), congenital (birth defect, developmental anomaly)
Chemicals	
	B. *Degenerations* (deposits) ⟶ necrosis (death) ⟶ scar; water, fat, pigments, ↓ lysis ⟶ resolution ↓ infection ⟶ abscess
Irradiation	
Genes	atrophy (decrease size)
	C. *Circulatory disturbances*
Nutrition	Hyperemia (stasis), ischemia, infarct, hemorrhage
	D. *Inflammation*
Bacteria	Vascular, cellular, proliferation (growth); repair
	E. *Growths* (tumor-like)
Viruses	Hypertrophy (increase in cell size), hyperplasia (increase in cell number), metaplasia (change in cell type)
Emotions	F. *Tumors*
	Benign (hamartoma), malignant
Others	

disturbances. They also include the inborn errors that result in metabolic disorders such as the inability of a cell to utilize a specific enzyme properly. In phenylketonuria there is a deficient enzyme which causes an amino acid to not be metabolized and, consequently, to build up in the blood stream. The PKU laboratory test in newborns can check for this inborn defect which if undetected can lead to mental retardation early in life. Agenesis and aplasia are terms used to describe the absence of a part or all of an organ to develop. For example, a person may be born without a kidney and still live. Dentally, many people have congenitally missing mandibular third molars. Malformations constitute an important part of oral pathology and more information will be given in another chapter.

Degenerative changes refer to metabolic disturbances and deteriorations of cells or the area immediately surrounding the cells. It is a state that may be irreversible leading to the death of the cell (necrosis). Microscopically within the cytoplasm of the cell one may see accumulation of water, fat, mucin, or pigments. For example, in alcoholic ingestion, cells of the liver swell with fat droplets which impair the function of the cell. This may be reversed by stopping the alcoholic intake, thereby returning the function of the cell to normal. However, if the injury is severe and the cell is overwhelmed, necrosis will be the end result. Necrosis refers to the death of tissue and, microscopically, is noted by changes in the nucleus such as the splitting apart of the nucleus. Without a nucleus to direct activities, the cell dies. The body resolves necrosis in many ways. Most commonly, the necrotic cells are localized and resorbed by other cells, with a scar replacing the area of necrosis. However, other possibilities exist. The necrotic cells may dissolve (lysis) and become liquefied. If the liquid is surrounded by epithelial cells, a cyst will remain. If the necrotic cells become infected secondarily, an abscess or collection of pus will result. Rather than being resorbed, the necrotic cells may become a focus for calcification and leave a hardened mass. In bone, the necrotic cells may become separated (sequestrated) from the sound bone cells.

Inactive cells or cells inflicted with a chronic metabolic deficiency may undergo atrophy. Atrophy refers to a decrease in the size of the cell compared to a normal cell. This wasting away of cells may ultimately be reflected in a decrease in the number of cells (numerical atrophy) as the degenerative process proceeds to necrosis of many of the atrophic cells.

On a clinical level, the category of degeneration is not used frequently, but the processes described here are seen often. For instance, an ulcer of the mouth has a necrotic surface. A tooth with deep decay may eventually have an abscess or cyst at the root end of the tooth. These are specific results of degenerative processes. But degenerative changes may be apparent in a more general manner. For example, the ill feeling or malaise that we have with a common cold is caused by degeneration in many cells throughout the body, particularly of the head, neck, and chest if it is an upper respiratory infection.

Circulatory disturbance is an important category of disease. Even under normal conditions there is a constant interplay of hyperemia (activity) and anemia (rest). Hyperemia refers to an increase in the blood supply; anemia, to a decrease in the number of red blood cells. By example, at rest there are capillaries in the lung that are without blood cells. Only a portion of the alveoli are at work. By contrast, during a brisk run, many more alveoli are used and more capillaries are filled with blood cells causing hyperemia.

In pathologic circumstances, there is also hyperemia. In active hyperemia there is an increased inflow of blood to an area. Passive hyperemia refers to a decreased outflow of blood with a stagnation of venous current. This stasis may lead to necrosis of tissues because of lack of oxygen to the site. Ischemia refers to the local deficiency of blood to an area. If the area involved is supplied by a single blood vessel, then the area will undergo ischemic necrosis or infarction and the area of necrosis will be called an infarct. The most common example is a myocardial infarction caused by an obstruction of blood flow from the coronary arteries to the heart muscle (heart attack).

Hemorrhage or bleeding is a circulatory disturbance caused by injury to capillaries, decrease in blood platelets, decrease in fibrinogen, and many other factors. The mechanism to prevent hemorrhage is clotting. If the inner lining of a blood vessel is damaged, a thrombus may form at the site of damage. Thrombosis is the formation of a plug within a blood vessel. The thrombus or clot is composed of red blood cells, platelets, and fibrin.

Blood clots are most common in veins, particularly those of the lower legs, where the superficial veins of the legs often become tortuous and bulge. The blood stagnates within them and injury is common. This may lead to the formation of a thrombus. Once formed, a thrombus is treated like foreign material and the body reacts to it in several ways. Certain cells may dissolve it and the lumen of the vessel will be patent again. Or other cells grow into the clot and bind it down to the wall so that it will not become free. Eventually new channels or capillaries are formed and in time blood can flow through the vessel again. Sometimes, however, the clot or a portion of it may dislodge from the site of its formation and be transported to a distant site where it can lodge in a smaller vessel. The detached clot is then termed an embolus or more specifically a thromboembolus. The detached and floating clot is the most common threat in patients following major surgery, because clots may form readily in legs that are immobile. However, there are other types of emboli, namely, air, bacteria, cells, fat, or foreign materials. Both the thrombus and emboli are significant because they can partly or completely occlude vessels and cause ischemia to a vital area. For instance,

a clot in a vessel to the brain could lead to apoplexy (a stroke). Besides a clot, a cerebrovascular accident (CVA) may be caused by hemorrhage into the brain tissue. Without oxygen, the brain cells quickly undergo liquefaction necrosis. Usually there is a loss of motor function and coordination corresponding to the area of necrosis. As the clot or hemorrhage is resolved, some function returns; however, those brain cells which underwent necrosis would not be replaced by brain cells but by scar tissue cells. Circulatory disturbance is a major category of disease which accounts for many diseases including heart disease, the major cause of death today.

Inflammation is a major category of disease. Through inflammation and immunology the host can cope with both living and nonliving foreign agents. Both involve complex interactions of blood-borne elements and cellular elements that are brought forth to combat the offending agent. Not only does the host respond in an overwhelming manner to the injurious agent, but it also sets the stage for repairing the injury by producing new cells rapidly (proliferation).

Repair of tissue is the replacement of the injured area with scar tissue (connective tissue cells). Regeneration is the replacement of damaged tissue with the same type of tissue that was damaged. For example, damaged heart muscle cannot regenerate and is replaced by scar tissue. On the other hand, surface epithelium or bone regenerates rapidly. However, if the destruction of tissue is extensive, even tissue with a good ability for regeneration will heal by repair (dense connective tissue).

Growth of tissue is another way the host can respond to injury. This proliferation of cells may or may not be associated with inflammation. The changes involved include hyperplasia, hypertrophy, and metaplasia. Hyperplasia is the increase in the number of normal cells of an organ or tissue with a consequent increase in size of the tissue. (Fig. 2.1). Hyperplasia can be physiologic, such as the response of glands to a demand for more secretion. Usually, how-

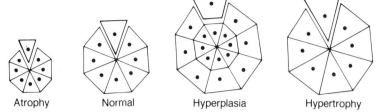

Figure 2.1. Schematic diagram of tissue and cellular changes. The dots represent nuclei within the cell.

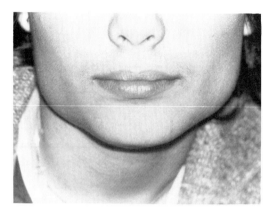

Figure 2.2. Hypertrophy of masseter muscles causing swellings at angles of the mandible.

ever, the increase in the number of cells is a protective mechanism against a constant source of irritation. The oral epithelium undergoes hyperplastic changes to injury which will be discussed under mucous membrane pathology in Chapter 6. Quite often, the underlying supporting tissue will undergo hyperplasia along with the surface tissue. An example of this is seen in denture hyperplasia caused by a poor fitting denture.

Hypertrophy (Fig. 2.1) is the increase in size of a tissue or organ caused by an increase in the size of the cells of the part involved. This is seen particularly in muscle fibers. For example, in a patient with heart failure, the heart muscles may undergo hypertrophy as a means of compensating for the original damage. Hypertrophy occurs physiologically in exercising of muscles and accounts for enlarged body contours. The masseter muscles may be prominent due to hypertrophy either ge-

netically or in individuals who constantly clench their teeth together (Fig. 2.2).

The opposite of hypertrophy is atrophy (Fig. 2.1). In a paraplegic, there is loss of nerve supply to the muscles of the legs and therefore loss of function. With loss of function, the muscle cells undergo atrophy. They decrease in size below normal and ultimately the whole muscle mass and leg become smaller. Atrophy can also be seen in the oral cavity. For instance, a defect in the hypoglossal nerve which innervates the tongue muscles will cause the tongue muscles to become atrophic. The muscles on the side affected will be shriveled. The tongue will not look full and will be flaccid (weak and soft) (Figs. 2.3 and 2.4).

Metaplasia is the microscopic change in which cells of one type are transformed or replaced by cells of another type that normally would not be located in the particular site. For instance, in smokers, the ciliated epithelium that lines bronchioles transforms into stratified squamous epithelium. This transformation is a protective mechanism in the sense that stratified squamous epithelium is more resistant to injury. However, the ciliated epithelium is itself a natural protective mechanism, so that metaplasia in this instance is an abnormal response. This same type of change is seen in ducts of accessory salivary glands in the oral cavity (Fig. 2.5).

Metaplasia is noted in the connective tissue cells as well as in the epithelial cells (Fig. 2.5). For example, bone or cartilage may form within connective tissue in an area that usually does not have bone or cartilage within it. The transformation of

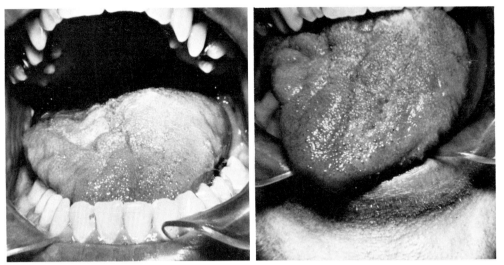

Figure 2.3. *Left*, hypoglossal nerve defect. Right side of tongue is atrophied and flaccid.
Figure 2.4. *Right*, hypoglossal nerve defect (same patient as in Figure 2.3). Tongue deviates to the affected side when protruded.

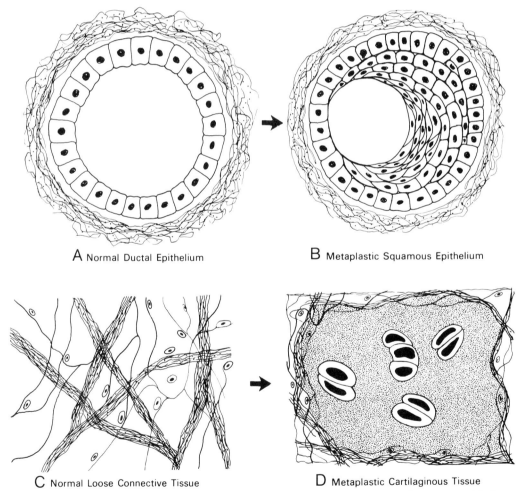

A Normal Ductal Epithelium

B Metaplastic Squamous Epithelium

C Normal Loose Connective Tissue

D Metaplastic Cartilaginous Tissue

Figure 2.5. Diagrammatic representation of metaplasia. *A* and *B*, metaplasia of ductular epithelium to stratified squamous epithelium. *C* and *D*, metaplasia of normal loose fibrous connective tissue to cartilaginous tissue.

normal connective tissue cells into the cells and substance comprising bone is metaplasia.

This concept of metaplasia is difficult to grasp, because it cannot be appreciated at the clinical level. Whereas the increase in cells of hyperplasia causes an increase in the overall size of a structure so as to produce a clinical lesion, the changes seen in metaplasia are microscopic only. For instance, a swelling on the gingiva is a hyperplastic response. However, on examining the tissue of this lesion by the microscope, one may see bone forming in the connective tissue (metaplasia). Metaplasia and pathologic hyperplasia contribute to cellular turnover and may predispose the tissues to neoplastic change.

Neoplasia is the last category to be considered. The term neoplasia refers to a new growth of tissue which arises from existing tissue but grows independently of it and at its own rate. This abnormal new tissue is called a neoplasm technically, but more commonly it is called a tumor. Strictly speaking, a tumor is any swelling of tissue and as such may represent a lesion that is developmental, inflammatory, or neoplastic. By common usage the word tumor has become synonymous with a neoplasm, specifically, cancer.

Clinically, a neoplasm may present as a swelling. Only by microscopic examination of the tissue can the nature of the lesion become known. By the cellular characteristics, the growth is designated as benign or malignant. Those neoplasms that resemble the tissue of origin in cellular details and in behavior are called benign. These are slow growing, localized lesions which may cause injury to the host by expansion against normal tissue or by releasing hormones.

By contrast, those neoplasms that present a marked difference in cellular details from the tissue of origin and are a threat

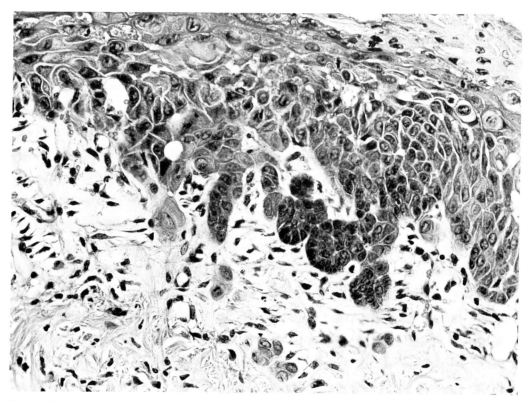

Figure 2.6. Squamous cell or epidermoid carcinoma. Atypical neoplastic epithelial cells extending and invading in clawlike extensions into underlying connective tissue.

to life or health because of their behavior are called malignant. The word cancer refers to any malignant neoplasm. Cancer of epithelial cells is a carcinoma. Cancer of connective tissue cells is a sarcoma. Cancers do not remain localized and can spread in many ways. The cells can grow in finger or claw-like projections and infiltrate the underlying tissue (Fig. 2.6).

Or the cells may spread by way of the lymph channels or blood stream. If a second growth of the malignancy occurs at the distant site, the cancer is said to have metastasized. Metastasis is a characteristic feature of malignancy. For example, a female patient may have a primary cancer of the breast. This cancer often spreads to the bones. Not infrequently one may see on the radiograph a radiolucency or dark shadow in the mandible near a tooth. On investigation, the tissue from this area of the jaw may reveal the same cancer cells that originated in the breast. The cancer in the jaw has grown at a distant site and is therefore a metastasis.

Neoplasia can occur anywhere in the body. Developing from different tissues in different areas, cancer is more than a hundred different diseases. In the oral cavity it is a serious disease because, despite the ease with which it could be diagnosed, the cure rate and survival rates are poor. Neoplasms of the oral cavity will be covered in another section.

In summary, there are numerous causes both known and unknown for disease, but the responses by the host are limited. Some agents may cause minimal injury while others may be overwhelming and cause severe damage. The extent of damage and the response depends on the resistance of the host. Given the same injury, each host will react differently; the injury may be slight to one but severe to another. The responses of any host to an injury as presented in this section may also be used at the clinical level. When one is contemplating a disease, it is convenient to ask what category of disease one has at hand. These categories are developmental, metabolic, inflammatory (infectious), hyperplastic, and neoplastic.

CHAPTER 3

Inflammation and Repair

The category of disease called inflammatory is extremely important in a discussion on oral pathology. Inflammation is a common, favorable response of the body to irritants or microorganisms. Without inflammation wounds would not heal, and bacteria and other organisms would flourish and eventually cause the death of the host. With inflammation the host has a nonspecific reactive process that not only walls off the area of injury but also sets into motion the process whereby the tissue may be healed.

The cause of the injury can be mechanical such as trauma, tear, laceration, etc.; it may be thermal or electrical and produce a burn; or it may be biological such as viral, bacterial, or fungal. Whatever the cause, cells at the site of injury are damaged, and chemicals from these cells set in motion the continuum of events called inflammation.

Inflammation is designated by the attachment of the suffix "itis," meaning inflammation of, to the name of the area that is affected. Thus, inflammation of the colon is colitis; of the veins, phlebitis; of the gingiva, gingivitis; of the pulp, pulpitis. Regardless of the location, the events of inflammation are the same.

The events seen in inflammation are complex and should be considered as an ever changing and dynamic picture. For convenience the components of the reaction are: damage to the tissues, a local change in circulation (alteration), infiltration of cells and fluid into the area (exudation), and the local proliferation of cells and growth of new tissue (granulation and repair).

Immediately following injury there is a brief moment in which the blood vessels in the area constrict. Test this by scratching the skin of the inside aspect of the wrist with a sharp point. You will observe that the line of the scratch blanches almost immediately due to the constriction of the blood vessels. Then the blood vessels, particularly the post capillary venules, dilate and become quite prominent (Fig. 3.1). This vascular change brings more blood to the area by both active and passive hyperemia. It also causes the flow of blood within the vessels to slow down (stasis). The red blood cells and the white blood cells move from the center of the venule to the edges (margination). Because of the vasodilation, there are gaps created between the endothelial cells. Lipid, salts and water leave in greater than normal amounts. Proteins, normally held back by intact endothelial cells, also leave the vessels. The red blood cells leave by a process called diapedesis, leaving in between the cells of the intact blood vessel. The more damage there is to the vessel, the greater will be the number of red blood cells (hemorrhage) in the injured area. Clinically, if the site of injury is observable, such as the scratch, a redness will appear and will increase over the hours as more blood comes to the area. Heat may also be noted and is due to the increase in the flow of blood to the area. The sluggish circulation is necessary for the next event which is the migration of cells (Fig. 3.2). Polymorphonuclear leukocytes or neutrophils are the first white blood cells called to the area by a chemical (chemotaxis), which is released by the injured cells. The summoned cells line up along the sides of the dilated blood vessels and by ameboid motion emigrate between endothelial cells into the injured area within a few hours

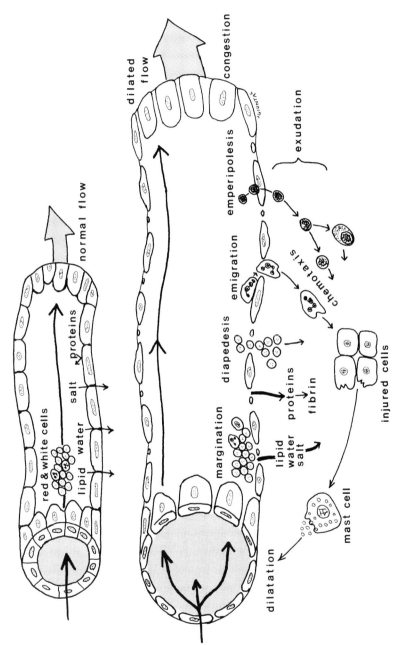

Figure 3.1. Diagram depicting particularly the early events of inflammation, vascular dilatation, fluid exchange, and cellular passage into the injured area.

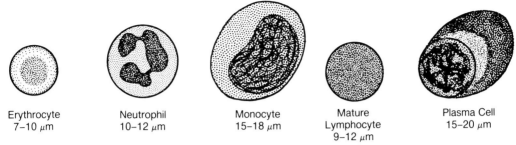

Erythrocyte
7–10 μm

Neutrophil
10–12 μm

Monocyte
15–18 μm

Mature
Lymphocyte
9–12 μm

Plasma Cell
15–20 μm

Figure 3.2. Diagrammatic representation of cells involved in inflammation, drawn to scale to illustrate relative size.

after the injury. Monocytes are the second white blood cell to emigrate. Lymphocytes usually enter much later but in some diseases, such as viral ones, they are the first to enter by crossing through the endothelial cells (emperipolesis).

Neutrophils are cells with many lobes of the nucleus which can assume multiple shapes and are therefore called polymorphonuclear cells. They are phagocytic cells, meaning that they can ingest microorganisms, other cells, like necrotic cells, and foreign matter. In the cytoplasm are numerous granules which stain on microscopic sections with neutral dyes and account for the name, neutrophil. These granules contain enzymes capable of digesting cellular tissue including bacteria.

Fluid in more than normal amounts (edema) also accumulates in the tissue. This fluid from the plasma of the blood contains fibrinogen. By the activation of the clotting mechanism in the tissues, fibrinogen is converted to fibrin, a large strandlike protein that forms a sponge-like mesh. The fibrin temporarily walls off the area and is capable of blocking drainage to lymphatic channels.

The fluid, protein and the cells outside of the blood vessels are called an exudate. The exudate accounts for the swelling which occurs clinically as, with time, more cells and fluid permeate into the area. With this accumulation there is pressure upon local nerve endings that may result in pain.

Certain factors are responsible for altering the permeability of the blood vessels and allowing extra fluid and cells to diffuse into the injured area. Histamine, derived from mast cells in tissue or basophils and platelets in blood, mediates the initial phase of permeability but its effect is short-lived. There are several vascular and tissue factors causing dilitation. Chemically antagonistic to the action of epinephrine, which constricts small vessels, they mediate the second phase. This phase lasts for several hours, during which time the neutrophils accumulate in the tissues and attempt to localize, destroy, and remove the agent as well as the damage.

Neutrophils are capable of ingesting and destroying some but not all bacteria. If the number of bacteria is such that the enzyme system of the neutrophil can digest them, then the area will soon be cleared of bacteria and neutrophils. Besides digesting bacteria and other small foreign particles, the lysosomes of neutrophils can dissolve the neutrophil itself if it dies, as well as liquefy local cells of the host and the insoluble fibrin wall that was laid down. If the number of bacteria are overwhelming or contain toxins to the neutrophils or the resistance of the host is decreased, neutrophils will accumulate, die, and in the process liquefy more host tissue and pus will form (suppuration). Pus is the liquefied material containing dead and dying neutrophils and host cell debris. When it is localized or walled off in a cavity it is called an abscess. It is usually eliminated by the body by drainage to an exterior surface such as skin or mucosa or diffuses by the blood or lymphatics where it is carried off for destruction elsewhere. A suppurative process may be seen in either acute or chronic inflammation.

The build-up of fluid, fibrin, and neutrophils is the hallmark of acute inflammation which, clinically speaking, usually lasts only for a short time (hours to days). Within hours, but more noticeable from 1 to 3 days, other cells begin to appear and to proliferate.

Macrophages, important in acute and chronic inflammation, appear after the neutrophils. Macrophages, also known as histiocytes, are derived from the white blood cell, the monocyte. They respond more slowly to chemicals liberated by injured cells (chemotaxis). They are also phagocytic cells but are larger and capable of ingesting larger particles. In fact, it is common to see an ingested neutrophil within the cytoplasm of a macrophage. In certain instances the cytoplasm of several macrophages merge with neighbors to form a large cell with multiple distinct nuclei, the foreign body giant cell. This type of cell can be seen in reactions to a wood splinter, to a suture, and to microorganisms such as fungi and the tubercle bacillus. Oftentimes, giant cells are seen in long-standing inflammation.

The prime function of the macrophage is to phagocytize foreign material, dead cells, and debris at the site of inflammation. Because of their time of appearance and function, they are considered the second line of defense. In most instances the neutrophils and macrophages can readily contain the injurious agent. However, if they fail, there is another system of cells called the reticuloendothelial system (RES) that can carry on. These cells resemble macrophages and are located scattered in connective tissue and particularly in the liver, the spleen, and lymph nodes.

The lymphocyte is another cell that appears later in the inflammatory process. This is a small cell with a densely stained round nucleus and very little cytoplasm. There are several types of lymphocytes whose prime function is to recognize foreign material (antigens) and to elaborate an immune response. Some of these cells are phagocytic and are capable of attaching themselves to an antigen. Other lymphocytes transform into plasma cells which serve to produce antibodies. Plasma cells have a nucleus, similar to the lymphocyte, but eccentrically located in a cytoplasm housing the machinery for producing the antibody. The antibody is expressed into the fluid surrounding the cells; it seeks out the foreign proteins and inactivates them by binding them to antigen-antibody complexes. These complexes themselves can elicit an inflammatory response.

Another cell that is involved in antigen-antibody responses, particularly relating to allergy, is the eosinophil. An eosinophil resembles a neutrophil with a lobulated nucleus but has prominent granules that stain red with the dye eosin. The granules contain enzymes capable of digesting antigen-antibody complexes. This may be the reason for the appearance of these cells in allergic diseases such as hay fever and contact allergies.

Fibroblasts and new capillaries also begin to appear within the first few days of the inflammatory response. The fibroblasts are young connective tissue cells that can produce collagen fibers. The new capillaries bud from existing capillaries in large numbers, increasing blood supply to the area. Collectively, the fibroblastic and new capillary response is called granulation tissue. The longer the granulation tissue remains, the more collagen fibers are formed and the greater amount of scar.

Both the macrocytic-lymphocytic infiltrate and the granulation tissue, a proliferation of cells and new tissue, are hallmarks of a chronic inflammatory response which clinically exists for an extended period (days to months or even years). If the injurious agent persists, then this response may linger without resolution and, with time, dense connective tissue (collagen) will replace the original tissue.

If the injurious agent is overcome, the inflammation will subside and the tissue will undergo repair. There are two types of repair. Restitution is the replacement of the injured area with the same tissue that preceded the inflammation. Repair with scarring (fibrosis) is the other form. A scar represents dense bundles of collagen fibers that have been produced from the granulation tissue to replace the injured tissue. At first the scar may appear red to the surface because of the increased capillary supply from the granulation tissue. But over many months these capillaries disappear and the avascular scar remains white due to the dense bundles of collagen. Thus the end of inflammation is heralded by a return of the tissue to its normal state or to a state of repair with a scar (Fig. 3.3).

An excellent example of the inflammatory response is seen in wound healing of ulcerations of the oral mucosa (Figs. 3.4–3.9). An ulcer is any break in the epithelial surface which exposes the underlying connective tissue. With this break, the energies of the local cells are involved in reuniting the surface. Wound healing takes place with the formation of abundant granulation tissue and epithelial proliferation. This is called healing by secondary intention because the wound edges are not approximated and because the inflammatory response must fill in the destroyed tissue with granulation tissue that ultimately will be replaced. This type of healing is seen in ulcers, tooth extractions, and bone fractures. If, on the other hand, the tissue is wounded but the edges are touching or are brought in continuity with sutures, that healing is by first intention and does not require the exuberant cellular response seen in ulcerations. Thus, there is less scarring when wounds are sutured.

In an ulcer there is activity at both the epithelial surface and deep within the underlying connective tissue. The destruction of the epithelial surface and some connective tissue initiates the inflammatory response (Fig. 3.10). If there is bleeding, a

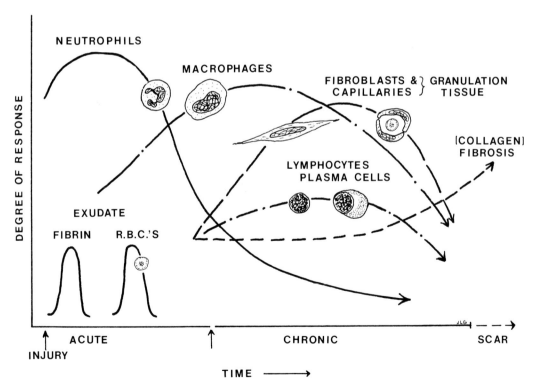

Figure 3.3. Schematic flow chart depicting events of the inflammatory response according to persistence of injury and time.

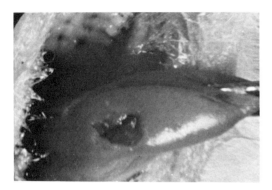

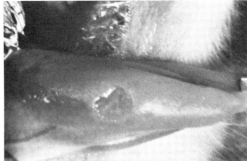

Figures 3.4.–3.9. Sequence following healing of experimental hamster.
Figure 3.4. Zero hours, fresh ulcer with bleeding.

Figure 3.6. One day, scab, complete, appears white.

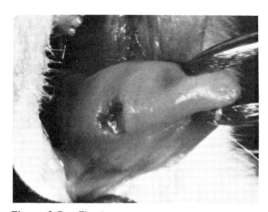

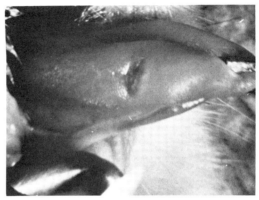

Figure 3.5. Five hours, early scab following clot.

Figure 3.7. Three days, ulcer contracted, rolled borders.

clot will soon form of fibrin and red blood cells. Within hours there is edema fluid, and neutrophils are seen in great numbers. The neutrophils begin to emigrate to the destroyed surface and ultimately build up the surface with a scab. The scab is composed of fibrin, red blood cells, and dead or dying neutrophils (Fig. 3.11). It is a necrotic plug and appears white or yellowish clinically. It serves to protect the connective tissue until the epithelium can cover it again. At the same time there is cellular activity in the connective tissue. Macrophages soon appear and begin to phagocytize the necrotic cells and debris along with the neutrophils. In about a day, fibroblasts and capillaries begin to proliferate. On the surface at this time, the epithelial cells at the margins of the ulcer pile up slightly and

begin to migrate toward the epithelium on the other margin. The epithelium extends itself between the scab and the tissue beneath it. In a matter of days when the epithelium meets with opposite margins at the center, the migration stops and the scab is cast off. After about 2 days there is abundant granulation tissue. The new capillaries and inflammatory response cover an area greater in width than the original ulceration and gives the tissue a reddened hue or halo surrounding the ulcer (Fig. 3.12). Just as the epithelium migrates and regenerates, the connective tissue and skeletal muscle regenerates in the connective tissue. The granulation tissue, which becomes infiltrated with chronic inflammatory cells, provides the vascularity with its nutrients so that new tissue can form. If the damage was not severe or long-stand-

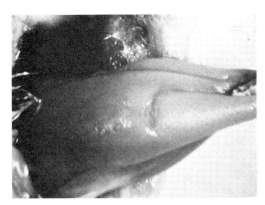

Figure 3.8. Seven days, epithelium healed, ulcer more contracted.

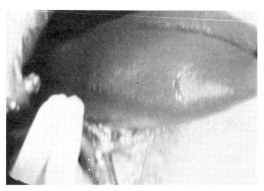

Figure 3.9. Fourteen days, only narrow defect remains, healing of connective tissue is continuing, contour of tongue is reestablished. At 21 days no evidence of an ulcer was seen.

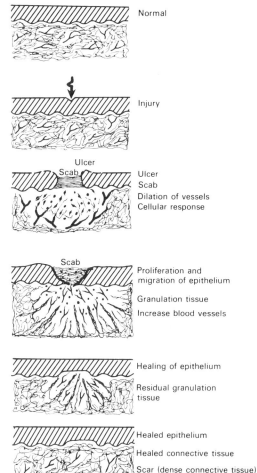

Figure 3.10. Reaction of mucosa to an injury that results in forming an ulcer. Schematic drawing depicting ulcer, scab formation, vascular and cellular response, formation of granulation tissue, proliferation, migration of epithelium, and healing by restitution of mucosal epithelium and connective tissue.

ing, not much fibrosis will occur—particularly in the oral mucosa. Rather the connective tissue will reform and muscle fibers and nerves will regenerate. Inflammatory cells and vascularity will subside and the tissue will be restored.

In healing where bone is involved, such as a socket site or removal of a lesion in the jaws, similar changes occur. The granulation tissue forms, In time, the fibroblasts from the granulation tissue transform into bone-forming cells and spicules of bone are laid down in the granulation tissue. Then calcium salts are incorporated into the new bone and mature bone results. This bone is reconstructed with time depending on the stresses it receives.

Inflammation is generally considered to be a favorable response, but there are oc-

casions when its consequences or continued existence is not so favorable. Inflammation of the cornea of the eye could lead to scarring and impairment of vision. That is why corticosteroid drops are used when the cornea is damaged. The corticosteroid as an anti-inflammatory agent diminishes the inflammatory response and consequent scarring. In the disease of poliomyelitis, which has been effectively abated by vaccination procedures, the complication of paralysis is a sign of inflammation that no longer ex-

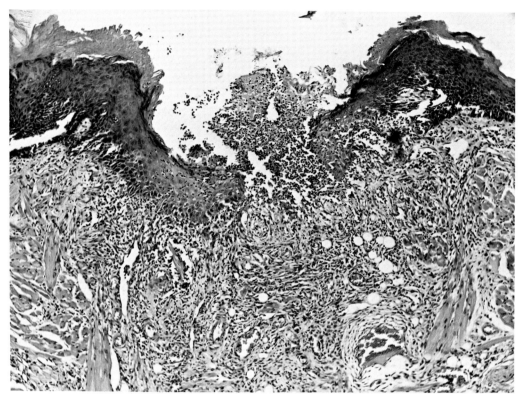

Figure 3.11. Healing experimental tongue ulcer, 4 days. Epithelium is migrating beneath scab. Margins of ulcer are rolled due to proliferating epithelium. Granulation tissue, rich in blood vessels and containing chronic inflammatory cells, is beginning to form new connective tissue and muscle.

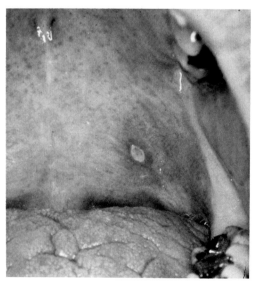

Figure 3.12. Ulcer on soft palate; aphthous stomatitis. Red halo surrounds clearly outlined oval white scab filling in ulceration.

ists. In poliomyelitis, important ganglion cells are infected by a virus and destroyed. Inflammation ensues and quickly heals the area. However, the area heals with scar tissue because the specialized nerve cells cannot regenerate. Thus, without these cells to complete the proper synapses, the muscles lack control and, because of disease, undergo atrophy.

An autoimmune response is a type of inflammatory response against the tissues of the host. In these circumstances there are antigen-antibody complexes formed against the host's tissue which is recognized as foreign. The complexes elicit an inflammatory response with all of the fluid and cells. Rheumatoid arthritis is an example of this phenomenon. The consequent attacks of inflammation account for the pain and immobility in the affected joints.

CHAPTER 4

Developmental Abnormalities

Developmental abnormalities represent those disturbances in the pattern of human growth leading to external or internal changes. Some are so minor as to be merely a variation from the normal (e.g. mucosal tag). Others are more severe (e.g. cleft palate, cyst). Still others are devastating (e.g. monstrosities).

There are intrinsic and extrinsic factors responsible for the abnormalities. Sometimes, both are active. For example, identical twins can appear to be the same at first, but differences in their environment or upbringing can make them appear different despite the identical genes. The genetically determined abnormalities are due to inheritance or to mutations of the genes acquired from elements in the environment.

A birth defect may arise from a spontaneous mutation or through some alteration of the environment during uterine life. Sometimes there are lethal injuries and the fetus is aborted or is born dead. Other times there may be less severe injuries. The injury may be caused by a lack of oxygen (hypoxia). This is the leading cause of cerebral palsy and mental retardation. Malnutrition, hormonal disturbances, and chemicals such as thalidomide all may cause malformations.

Congenital malformations are those developmental anomalies present at birth. Some disturbances, however, are determined in utero yet they manifest later in life. Others may develop after birth and show up later in life.

Many of the developmental disturbances of the head and neck are minor, causing little or no disability. However, even two or three minor variations or malformations found in the head and neck (oral cavity) may be significant. They may be part of a syndrome (a set of symptoms or signs occurring together) which may be part of a more serious malformation. This book will refer to only a few syndromes. There are several excellent texts enumerating and discussing them.

An example in which there is a known relationship of cause and effect is the injury caused by the virus of german measles (rubella) to babies. A pregnant woman, getting the disease for the first time during the first trimester, may deliver a baby with many malformations. Again, there are many possibilities of damage depending on the timing of the insult. The fetus may die when it is incompatible with life. There may be severe malformations such as cataracts and congenital heart disease. Or there may be minimal damage such as enamel hypoplasia of the deciduous teeth and delayed eruption of the teeth.

The following is a presentation of developmental abnormalities of the soft tissue, jaws, and teeth.

SOFT TISSUE ABNORMALITIES

Cleft lip and cleft palate represent failures of fusion of islands of tissue during development. They are common in occurrence since 1 in 700 babies are born with one or the other, or both. More males are affected than females.

Cleft lip occurs on either side of the midline in the area corresponding to the maxillary lateral incisor and cuspid region. Most commonly it is unilateral with the left side being involved more often than the right (Fig. 4.1). However, both sides may be affected in which case the condition is bilateral and, because of the resemblance to the lip of the rabbit, may be referred to as a harelip. The cleft may be complete extending to the base of the nose or incomplete presenting as an indentation of the upper lip. It occurs between 4–7 weeks in utero which corresponds to the time the lip normally develops. Because of this specific time of development, cleft lip may occur independently of cleft palate. However, both cleft lip and cleft palate may occur together.

Cleft palate results from a failure of fusion of the developing palatine processes and premaxillary processes. It can vary in severity depending on the extent of the cleft from the alveolar ridge to the end of the soft palate. The variations seen reflect the sequence of development of the palate which begins in utero at 8 weeks in the premaxillary region and ends at 12 weeks at the uvula of the soft palate. Thus, if the etiologic factor were at work from the 8th week, the cleft would occur anteriorly to posteriorly including the alveolus, hard palate, soft palate and uvula, resulting in a gross and serious defect. On the other hand, if the cause were acting near the end of the developing period (11th week), the cleft would be seen only in the posterior soft palate resulting in a partial cleft or merely a bifid uvula (Fig. 4.2), a minor and innocuous defect that requires no treatment.

The cause of cleft lip and cleft palate is not definitely known. However, present theories favor both genetic and environmental factors. Treatment of the clefts is by surgical or mechanical closure. Usually teams of specialists from many disciplines work closely together to treat these young patients and to advise the parents.

Congenital lip pits are depressions on the lower lip which are rarely seen. The cause is unknown. No treatment is required.

Commissural lip pits are indentations which occur at the corners of the mouth.

Double lip is a pendulous fold of excess tissue on the inner aspect of the upper lip, usually seen on smiling. This can be surgically removed.

Macroglossia refers to an enlargement of the tongue. It may be developmental in origin, due to a hypertrophy of the tongue muscle. Because the tongue is large, it pushes against the teeth and indentations can be created on the lateral borders of the tongue, yielding a scalloped appearance (Fig. 4.3). Macroglossia is seen in the disease of mongolism, a genetic disease with many other developmental disturbances.

Macroglossia may also be acquired. Besides being developmental, enlarged tongues can be seen because of tumors, inflammation, and hormonal changes (cretinism, acromegaly). Depending upon its severity and potential to cause other problems within the oral cavity, the enlarged tongue may be reduced to size by surgery.

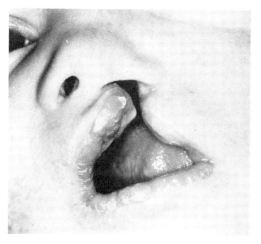

Figure 4.1. Complete cleft lip, unilateral.

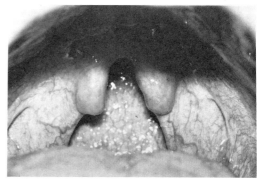

Figure 4.2. Partial cleft, soft palate, bifid uvula.

Microglossia refers to a small tongue. It is extremely rare. In hemiatrophy of the tongue, half of the tongue would be small. The cause may be a defect in the cranial nerve (hypoglossal) that innervates the tongue muscles. Without stimulation the tongue muscles atrophy and the body of the tongue becomes smaller. In this instance the defect in the tongue reflects damage elsewhere.

Ankyloglossia (tongue-tie) refers to the partial or complete attachment of the tongue to the floor of the mouth (Fig. 4.4). The lingual frenum is attached too far for-ward and may be seen in various positions, the most severe being at the tip of the tongue. Mobility of the tongue may be hampered, and patients cannot touch the hard palate when the mouth is opened. Speech may be impaired. Mild cases require no treatment, and severe cases can be treated successfully with surgical removal of the misplaced frenum.

Bifid tongue (forked tongue) represents the rare failure of fusion of the lateral halves of the tongue. It is seen in the midline at the tip as a notch (Fig. 4.5). Usually, no treatment is required.

Central papillary atrophy of the tongue (Fig. 4.6), previously called median rhomboid glossitis, is an ovoid or rhomboidal rashlike area in the midline of the dorsum of the tongue anterior to the circumvallate

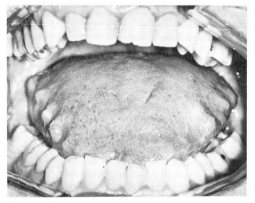

Figure 4.3. Macroglossia, scalloped borders of tongue correspond to embrasure spaces of teeth and are composed of tongue tissue.

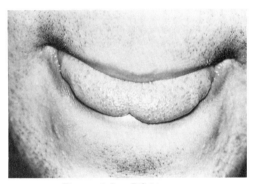

Figure 4.5. Bifid tongue.

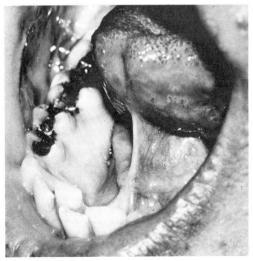

Figure 4.4. Ankyloglossia, broad lingual frenum attached near tip of tongue. Tongue is fully extended toward palate.

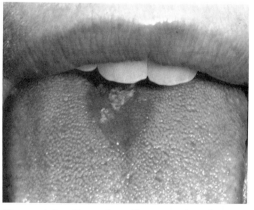

Figure 4.6. Central papillary atrophy of tongue (median rhomboid glossitis). This was due to *Candida albicans* infection. It disappeared with mycostatin treatment.

papillae occuring in 1% of the population. The filiform papillae are atrophic yielding a reddened zone, which may be flat or raised. Sometimes there are superimposed white lesions that may be scraped away. Originally, it was thought that the lesion was developmental resulting from the persistence of the tuberculum impar of the tongue, not being covered by the lateral halves of the tongue. However, it is rare to find this lesion in children. There is an association of this lesion with a fungus, *Candida albicans*, so that it may be an inflammatory process secondary to candidiasis (Fig. 4.7). Interestingly, *C. albicans* is a normal inhabitant of the oral mucosa and has been cultured in greater numbers at that site even in normal appearing tongues. Perhaps a change in the oral environment, triggered by a decrease in the immune response, allows the organism to flourish and cause the central atrophy. Smears of the lesions and biopsies yield the *Candida* organism. Antifungal medications can cause the lesion to disappear. However, because it may recur, treatment is used primarily for symptomatic lesions. Central papillary atrophy is a nuisance disease and is not a cancer, a fear of many patients.

Fissured or furrowed tongue is a common condition in which deep grooves occur in the dorsal surface of the tongue (Fig. 4.8). The fissures, resembling brain tissue, may

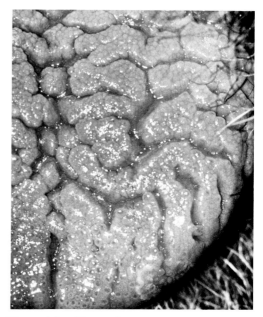

Figure 4.8. Fissured tongue, with deep grooves or crypts.

be mild or severe and seem to deepen with age. In some instances food and debris may lodge in the furrows and cause irritation with symptoms. In most cases there are no symptoms and no treatment is required. Fissured tongue may be acquired since it appears at older ages and is rarely seen in children.

Geographic tongue is an interesting condition that frequently occurs along with fissured tongue (Fig. 4.9). It is a common entity characterized by a loss of the filiform or white papillae in one or multiple areas of any surface of the tongue, particularly the dorsum. Red patchy areas are usually surrounded by a grayish white zone corresponding to the normal papillae with a pile up of some of the desquamated papillae. For this reason geographic tongue is considered as a white lesion. The rashlike areas assume many shapes, some of which resemble known geographic areas. Moreover, each time it is observed there is a different area with a different shape because one area heals as new papillae grow while another area loses the papillae. Thus other names have been ascribed, i.e. wandering rash, glossitis areata migrans. Because the nor-

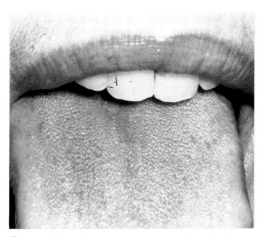

Figure 4.7. Normal tongue of patient in Figure 4.6 2 weeks posttreatment.

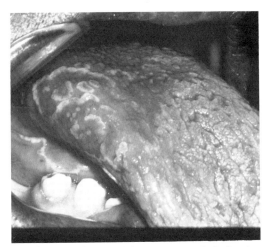

Figure 4.9. Geographic tongue and similar lesions (stomatitis migrans) of the adjacent floor of the mouth.

and do not desquamate or shed normally. Essentially the "hair" on the tongue is longer, particularly on the middorsal surface although the lateral borders may be involved (Fig. 4.11). The color can vary

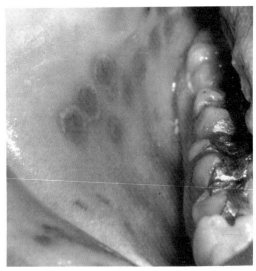

Figure 4.10. Stomatitis migrans of the buccal mucosa in patient with geographic tongue. The lesions are ringlike with red centers and raised white border.

mal protective papillae are lost, the atrophic areas may be irritated, inflamed and sensitive to certain foods. Usually, however, there are no symptoms and it is discovered on examination or by self-observation. The patient who does observe it may fear cancer and should be reassured that it is not significant and is not cancer. The true etiology of geographic tongue is obscure. There is a strong emotional component, and therefore it may be of psychosomatic origin. It has been noted in association with the common cold suggesting decreased immunity as a factor. This condition can recur. Lesions similar to geographic tongue may be seen in locations of the mucosa besides the tongue with or without the presence of tongue lesions. This ectopic geographic tongue has been called stomatitis migrans (Fig. 4.10). It seems to be psychosomatic in origin and interestingly, like geographic tongue and central papillary atrophy, microscopically resembles psoriasis, a recognized psychosomatic disease of the skin. These lesions also may change, may disappear and may recur. No specific treatment beyond diagnosis and reassurance is needed.

Hairy tongue is a condition, not specifically developmental, in which the filiform papillae elongate or undergo hypertrophy

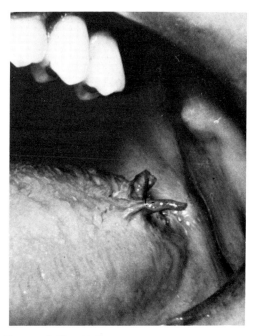

Figure 4.11. Hairy tongue, brown stain. Extremely long filiform papillae. Patient was a heavy smoker.

from white to brown or black or other colors depending on what produces the pigment. One cause is thought to be dehydration. For instance, in the common cold, the tongue appears white and "coated." Poor oral hygiene may be another factor. Patients on antibiotics may get a black hairy tongue (lingua nigra) due to the overgrowth of pigment-producing bacteria that are allowed to grow in excess because the normal oral bacterial flora is upset (Fig. 4.12). The condition disappears after stopping the antibiotic. The colors seen in hairy tongue, or even in the normal tongue, may be influenced by pigments in coffee, tea, tobacco, candy, and lozenges. Hairy tongue is benign. Better hygiene, such as brushing or scraping the tongue, may be suggested. Otherwise no treatment is required.

White sponge nevus is a hereditary disease in which several siblings and members of the same family exhibit excess folds of white, soft, spongy tissue. It can be seen anywhere on the mucosa but is common on the buccal mucosa and the lateral borders of the tongue. Mistaken for leukoplakia, it is similar to leukoedema. Adequate family history of the condition and biopsy confirms the diagnosis. No treatment is required.

Fordyce's granules or spots (Fordyce's disease) is not a disease but a developmental condition that is extremely common, occurring in 80% of the population. Fordyce's spots are multiple, small, yellow-white, submucosal papules that represent ectopic sebaceous glands without hair follicles. They can occur anywhere on the mucosa but are most commonly seen on the mucosal surface of the lips and on the buccal mucosa on each side (Figs. 1.10 and 1.14). When they occur in other locations, or as single glands, the diagnosis is not so obvious (Fig. 4.13). They lie just beneath the mucosa and become more visible as the mucosa is stretched. They can vary greatly in number and may be so clustered in some patients that they evoke concern. They are of no clinical significance. They do not represent cancer. No treatment is required.

Fibromatosis gingivae (hereditary gingival fibromatosis) is a diffuse enlargement of the gingivae characterized by a growth in the connective tissue component (Fig. 4.14). It is inherited as a dominant trait and may be associated with other abnormalities. The gingivae are firm, normal in color, and may cover the crown of the teeth. Treatment is surgical removal of the excess tissue.

Tori are innocuous hard mucosal swell-

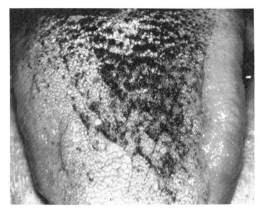

Figure 4.12. Black hairy tongue in 65-year-old who was taking penicillin for a tooth abscess. The filiform papillae are elongated and covered with chromophilic bacteria.

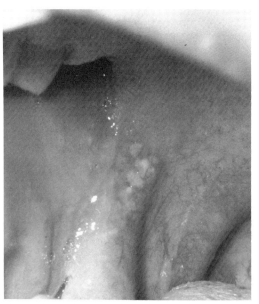

Figure 4.13. Fordyce's glands on retromolar pad. They are yellow submucosal clusters.

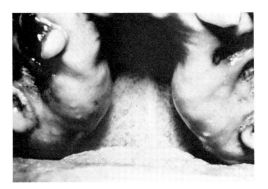

Figure 4.14. Gingival fibromatosis.

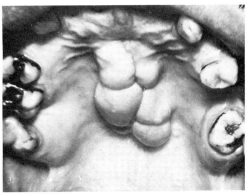

Figure 4.15. Torus palatinus, multiple bone projections in the midline of the hard palate covered by mucosa. Mucosa is exposed to traumatic insults.

ings which protrude from the jaws. They represent an excess of normal bone formation, appear radiopaque and can occur in various sites. In the midline of the hard palate one can occur as a single or multiple nodular mass and is termed a torus palatinus (Figs. 1.16 and 4.15). In the mandible they usually occur as bilateral whitened masses lingual to the roots of the premolar teeth and are called tori mandibularis (Figs. 4.16 and 4.17). Similar projections of bone may appear on the labial or buccal surface of either the maxillary or mandibular alveolar ridges and are termed exostoses (bone outside of bone) (Figs. 1.16 and 4.18). Tori are more common in females. Usually no treatment is required. If they interfere with dentures, other prostheses, or speech, they can be removed surgically.

DEVELOPMENTAL ABNORMALITIES OF JAWS

Macrognathia refers to a large jaw. In the mandible this would result in a protrusion (class III, Angle) with the chin being very prominent. It may be a congenital development which can be corrected by surgery. It may also be acquired through disease. In acromegaly, the patients have a tumor of the pituitary gland. This promotes continued growth at specific sites such as the fingers and the jaw bone of the mandible.

Micrognathia refers to a small jaw, usually involving the mandible. The chin may be severely receded or even absent (Fig. 4.19). The resulting prominence of the nose

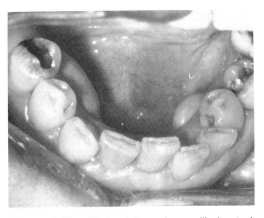

Figure 4.16. Bilateral lingual mandibular tori. Firm swellings behind bicuspid teeth.

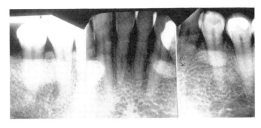

Figure 4.17. Lingual tori radiographically noted as opaque oval areas lingual to bicuspids. Same patient as Figure 4.16).

and upper lip has promoted the term "bird face," The cause is developmental or acquired. Injury to the condyle by trauma at birth or infection about the ears may cause the growth center of the condyle to be affected. This may be corrected by surgery.

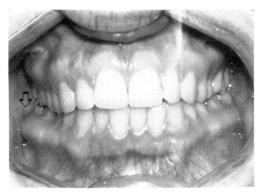

Figure 4.18. Bilateral shelflike exostoses (*arrow*) of posterior mandible in a young woman. Gingivae were normal.

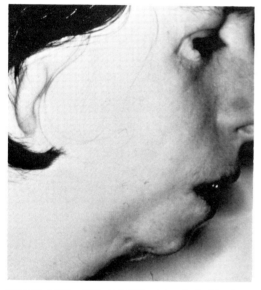

Figure 4.19. Micrognathia, retruded chin, lowset, malformed ear and malformed eye in patient with Treacher Collins syndrome.

If the jaws develop incorrectly, there may be crowding of teeth and the jaws may fail to approximate each other so that the teeth do not meet properly or are in poor position for function or esthetics.

There are several disorders that affect the jaws as well as other areas. Some of these have a specific set of signs or symptoms associated with them and are called syndromes. An example, is Pierre Robin's syndrome. These children are born with severe micrognathia of the mandible,

drooping of the tongue, and cleft palate. Other defects such as deformities of the ear may also be present. Another example is the Treacher Collins syndrome (Fig. 4.19).

DEVELOPMENTAL DISTURBANCES OF THE TEETH

During the formation of a tooth, the tooth bud may be disturbed so that any or all of the components of the tooth are affected. The cause may be local, systemic, or hereditary. The clinical manifestation will vary depending on the stage of development, the insult, and the length of time it occurs. The formative cells are very sensitive. Insults may affect these cells until the tooth is calcified. There may be variations in number, size, shape, position, eruption, and structure. The disorder may appear independently or in association with some other condition.

If the tooth germ fails to initiate, *anodontia* occurs. Anodontia refers to the failure of teeth to appear or develop. Absolute anodontia or the failure of all teeth to develop is extremely rare. However, it can be seen in a hereditary disease called ectodermal dysplasia. In this condition, which involves mainly males, structures derived from ectoderm (from which the tooth is derived) are involved. These individuals are missing hair, sweat glands, sebaceous glands, and teeth—both primary and permanent. They may have complete or partial anodontia.

Partial anodontia is more common in the general population. Perhaps representing an evolutionary sign, the most common missing tooth is the mandibular third molar. The next most common congenitally missing tooth is the maxillary lateral incisor (Fig. 4.20).

Cleidocranial dysplasia is an interesting condition in which the clavicle fails to develop and the cranial sutures fail to close on time so that the eyes are wide apart (hypertelorism). In addition the patients may show a clinical partial anodontia due to faulty eruption. However, radiography reveals multiple impacted teeth and extra teeth.

Extra teeth or those that develop in excess of a normal complement are called supernumerary or accessory teeth. They can occur in either jaw but are seen most frequently in the maxilla in the midline of the anterior teeth and distal to the molar teeth. When the extra tooth occurs between the maxillary central incisors, it is called a mesiodens (Figs. 4.21 and 4.22). These teeth usually are small (microdontia), are peg-shaped, and do not resemble the teeth normal to the site. However, some supernumerary teeth may mimic very closely a normal tooth (Fig. 4.23). They may erupt or remain embedded in tissue or impacted in bone. A mesiodens that is impacted can

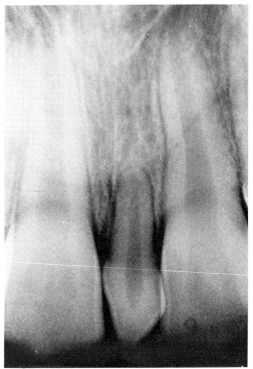

Figure 4.22. Radiograph of mesiodens. Note small size (microdontia).

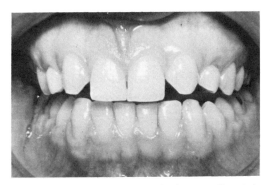

Figure 4.20. Congenitally missing maxillary lateral incisors.

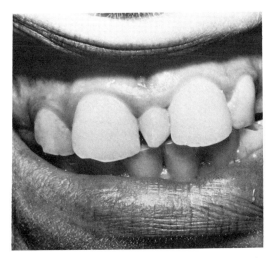

Figure 4.21. Mesiodens, supernumerary tooth between maxillary central incisors.

cause a diastema or spacing between the maxillary central incisors. Supernumerary teeth may cause crowding of the normal teeth and may delay the eruption of permanent teeth. Treatment is surgical removal.

Occasionally and rarely a newborn may have a tooth that erupts prior to birth (natal) or soon after birth (neonatal). Before removing them, they must be distinguished from a prematurely erupted primary tooth.

Macrodontia refers to a large tooth (Fig. 4.24). Some teeth may be quite large in width or height when compared to sizes that are known for normal teeth. Other teeth may be large because of some developmental defect other than just size.

Gemination results in a large tooth because a single tooth germ attempts to form two teeth (Figs. 4.25–4.27). This twinning usually results in partial or completely separated crowns attached to a single root with one canal.

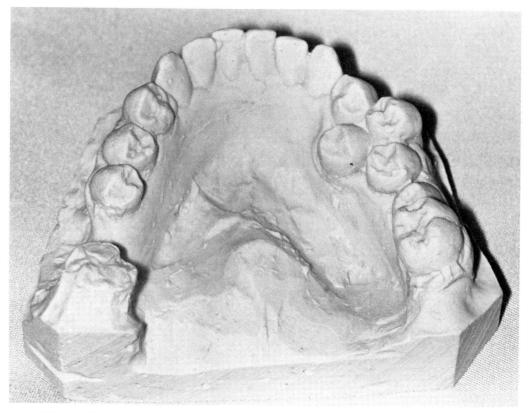

Figure 4.23. Study model showing several supernumerary bicuspid teeth.

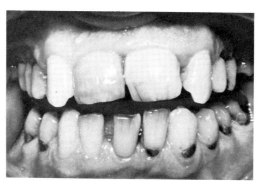

Figure 4.24. Macrodontia of central incisors. Lateral incisors were missing.

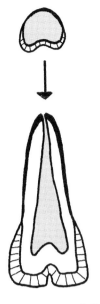

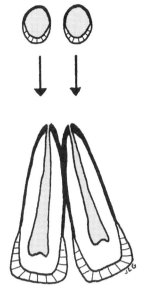

GEMINATION

one bud
one tooth
one canal

FUSION

two buds
two teeth
dentin union

CONCRESCENCE

two buds
two teeth
cementum union

Figure 4.25. Diagrams of gemination, fusion and concrescence. All three present clinically as macrodontia.

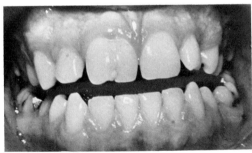

Figure 4.26. Gemination. The maxillary right central incisor appears to be two teeth (macrodontia). The lateral incisor is present.

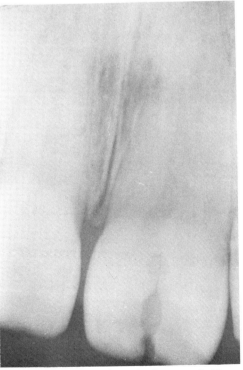

Figure 4.27. X-ray of gemination seen in Figure 4.26. Note two pulp chambers and single root canal.

Fusion results in formation of one tooth from two separate tooth germs. This usually results in macrodontia with a large crown composed of the joined crowns (Fig. 4.28) and joined roots usually with two root canals (Fig. 4.29). Fusion and gemination may be difficult to distinguish. A count of teeth present may be helpful since in fusion there should be one tooth missing.

Dens in dente means a tooth within a tooth. This describes the radiographic appearance of a dental anomaly caused by the invagination of the enamel into a deep groove in a tooth, frequently seen in the lingual pit area of the maxillary lateral incisor (Fig. 4.30). Because debris settles in the invagination, these teeth are prone to undetected decay, and periapical inflammation may be the first indication of the process.

Dilaceration (Fig. 4.31) refers to an abnormal angulation of the root with reference to the long axis of the crown. Usually it is very sharp and almost at a right angle. Trauma may be a factor so that the crown is displaced and a twist or bend results in the root that develops after the trauma. Dilaceration creates a problem on extraction of the tooth.

There may be disturbances in the position of teeth. Inadequate space for teeth results in crowding. These irregularities are

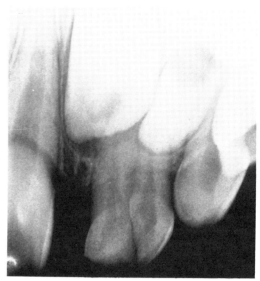

Figure 4.29. Radiograph showing fusion of deciduous central and lateral incisors. Note the separate root canals.

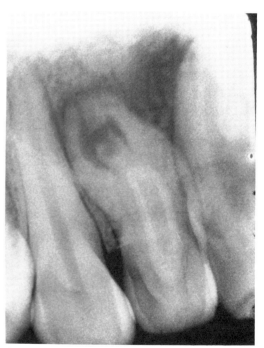

Figure 4.30. Dens in dente of maxillary lateral incisor associated with periapical radiolucency.

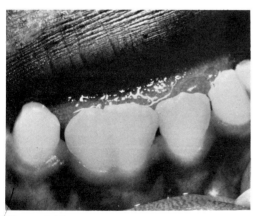

Figure 4.28. Fusion of mandibular right central and lateral incisor, creating a large tooth (macrodontia).

common. Some teeth may be completely rotated so that the buccal cusp is toward the lingual or palatal side. Other teeth may be transposed such that two teeth may

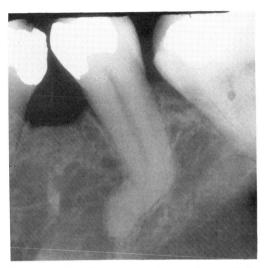

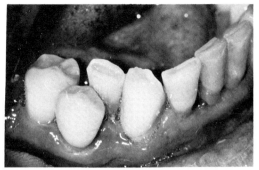

Figure 4.32. Transposition of mandibular right lateral incisor and cuspid teeth.

Figure 4.31. Dilaceration of root of mandibular bicuspid.

seem to have changed positions (Fig. 4.32). Or teeth may erupt in an abnormal position.

Although the pattern of eruption of teeth is normally quite variable in that no two individual patterns are alike, there are times in which the eruption may be premature or delayed. The cause for this is usually obscure; however, in some instances it can be related to certain events or systemic influences. Trauma with the loss of a primary tooth may cause the early eruption of the corresponding permanent tooth. In hyperthyroidism the teeth often erupt prematurely. Conversely, in the disease of hypothyroidism, with diminished metabolic activity, the eruption of the teeth is usually delayed. An impacted tooth represents an eruption pattern that is remarkably delayed.

ENAMEL HYPOPLASIA

If the ameloblasts are damaged during the period of tooth formation in which they are forming enamel matrix, the tooth will have defects in its form or shape. Enamel hypoplasia is the term used for the incomplete or defective formation of the enamel with resulting gross defects or change in form. Enamel hypoplasia may involve the primary and permanent dentition. It is quite common and occurs in about 10% of the population.

Clinically, there is a wide variation of appearances. Hypoplasia may appear as small pits, as rows of horizontal grooves or pits, or simply as missing enamel. If the insult was systemic, the hypoplasia involves the contralateral teeth with a pattern that corresponds to the time during which the teeth were forming. Because teeth follow a specific incremental development, the time of injury can be determined. For example, in permanent teeth, the majority of cases of hypoplasias occurs between 1 and 10 months of age. During this time, the crowns that are developing and that would show defects are the first molars, the incisors (except the maxillary laterals), and the canines. If the maxillary lateral incisors and the premolars are involved, the timing of the insult occurred between 11 and 34 months. Thus enamel hypoplasia provides a permanent record of an injury that occurred at a specific time. If the injury was of short duration the pits, grooves, or lines will involve only a narrow portion of the teeth. On the other hand, an extended period of injury will result in more tooth structure being defective and there may be a broad band that results (Figs. 4.33 and 4.34). Two bands, one at the incisal third and one at the cervical third of an incisor, for example, indicate two separate periods of injury (Fig. 4.35).

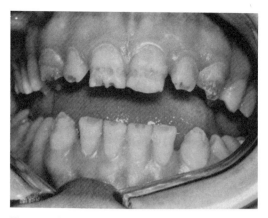

Figure 4.33. Systemic (environmental) hypoplasia, 17-year-old. The first molars, central and lateral incisors and canines show hypoplasia of the incisal third corresponding to the timing of matrix formation of these teeth. The hypoplasia is chronic because the patient was ill from birth through 18 months.

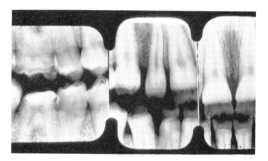

Figure 4.34. Radiographs of teeth with systemic (environmental) hypoplasia due to continuous respiratory infections from birth through 18 months of age. The bicuspids are not affected. Same patient as Figure 4.33.

There are various factors, known and unknown, that can injure the ameloblasts and cause hypoplasia. Nutritional deficiencies of vitamins A, C, and D can result in systemic hypoplasia. Patients with a history of rickets (vitamin D deficiency) often display severe hypoplasia. Diseases associated with high fevers, particularly measles and chickenpox, cause horizontal pitting. These pits accumulate debris and bacteria which can stain a deep brown.

Another cause of hypoplasia is congenital syphilis. In untreated pregnant women in-fected with syphilis, the causative spirochete invades the fetus after the 16th week and the tooth germs may be affected. In some of these children characteristic changes (stigmata) may be seen in the permanent anterior teeth and/or posterior teeth. Essentially, there is a reduction in the mesiodistal dimension of the teeth affected (Fig. 4.36). The anterior maxillary incisors are narrowed at the incisal third. The central incisors may resemble a screwdriver, may have a central notch, and are called Hutchinson's incisors after the physician who first attributed the change to syphilis. The lateral incisors usually are conical and are called peg-laterals. The first molar teeth are narrowed and may have numerous rounded cuspal structures on the occlusal surface. Resembling a mulberry, these teeth are called mulberry molars. Although these types of hypoplastic teeth are frequently associated with congenital syphilis, similar changes may be seen without such a history and more information would be required before the definitive association is made. For instance, peg-laterals, an example of microdontia and hypoplasia, are commonly seen but the cause is usually unknown.

Hypocalcemia is a decrease in calcium and can cause pitting of the teeth. This may be seen in the disease of hypoparathy-

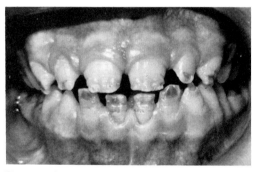

Figure 4.35. Systemic enamel hypoplasia. The broad areas with less enamel from incisal edges to junction of middle third indicate the child was ill enough to damage ameloblasts from birth through about 18 months. The separate linear defect in the middle third corresponds to tonsillitis at about 2½ years of age.

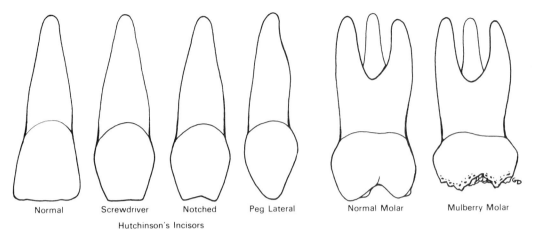

Normal — Screwdriver — Notched — Peg Lateral — Normal Molar — Mulberry Molar

Hutchinson's Incisors

Figure 4.36. Changes noted in teeth in patients with congenital syphilis. Basic change is hypoplasia with a loss of tooth structure in the mesiodistal diameter at the incisal or occlusal third of the teeth.

roidism as well as in vitamin D deficiency. The changes are the same as those seen in systemic hypoplasia.

Birth injury or premature delivery may cause a definite horizontal or mesiodistal defect seen as a line. This neonatal line is usually seen at the gingival third of the primary incisors and the tips of the first permanent molars.

When local factors are responsible the condition is called Turner's hypoplasia. Usually only one tooth is involved and this can be called a Turner's tooth (Fig. 4.37). There is not a symmetrical pattern and the time of injury is reflected on only the tooth involved, usually the permanent maxillary incisors or the premolars. The cause is trauma to the primary tooth or infection about the root of a primary tooth that affects the developing crown of the permanent tooth.

Chemicals may cause hypoplastic defects. Excessive amounts of fluoride can produce mottled enamel; the condition is called dental fluorosis (Fig. 4.38). Mottling is the discoloration of the enamel in irregular areas. There are two types of defects that can be noted, and the severity of the defects increases as the fluoride concentration increases. There may be white flecks or opacities (hypocalcification), pitting with loss of normal shape (hypoplasia), or

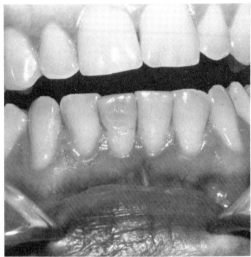

Figure 4.37. Turner's hypoplasia of mandibular right central incisor. Note horizontal indented line in middle of tooth.

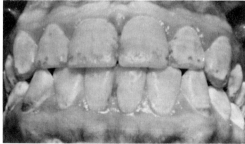

Figure 4.38. Dental fluorosis, mottled enamel. White varigated pattern of teeth is due to excessive quantities of fluorine in natural drinking water.

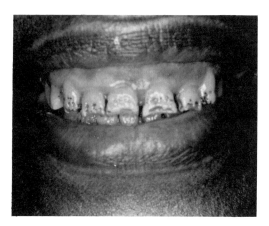

Figure 4.39. Severe dental fluorosis. Pitted hypoplastic defects due to high concentrations of fluorine in drinking water.

both (Fig. 4.39). The spots are white on eruption, but with time they acquire the brown stain that characterizes mottled enamel. The optimal level of fluoride in drinking water is considered one part per million because below that level there is little benefit in decreasing decay and above that level the dental fluorosis becomes prominent. Thus in communities with natural fluoride in the drinking water at five parts per million, teeth have little decay but may be severely mottled.

Probably the most common cause of hypoplasia is idiopathic, a term meaning cause unknown.

ENAMEL OPACITIES (HYPOCALCIFICATION)

Enamel opacities are white opaque spots that appear in permanent and primary teeth (Fig. 4.40). These are common and may be seen in 25% of the population. The maxillary central incisors are the teeth most commonly involved. Local or systemic factors similar to those in enamel hypoplasia are responsible. In this condition, however, the factor injures the tooth germ during the calcification stage. Thus, the defect is represented as a white spot because of the decrease of calcium at that time of injury. The shape and form of the teeth are normal in enamel opacities. It is likely, though, that a tooth may exhibit both

enamel opacities and hypoplastic defects so that, at times, the specific entities may be difficult to distinguish.

There are hereditary disturbances of the teeth which can affect the enamel, dentin, or pulp. The most common are those affecting the enamel and dentin.

Amelogenesis imperfecta or hereditary brown teeth is an inherited defect in the enamel featuring hypocalcification or hypoplasia of the enamel. The dentin and pulp are normal. Both the primary and the permanent teeth are affected. Incidence of the disease is 1 in 15,000 individuals. Many patterns of inheritance have been noted. Some are autosomal dominant, some recessive, some X-linked so that the number of individuals affected in a family can be variable. A family history for the trait may reveal that several members of a family in several generations have the disease. The gene defect causes the enamel to be hypocalcified or hypoplastic. Clinically, there may be a variation with pits, grooves, and defects occurring in horizontal or vertical patterns with no relationship to chronologic development. The most common type is the hypocalcified variety in which the teeth are originally normal in thickness, brown, friable, and soft. Calculus may build up heavily on the defects that occur as the

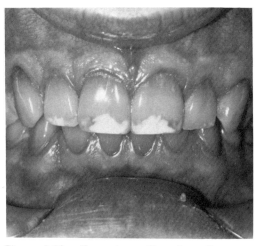

Figure 4.40. Enamel opacities of maxillary central incisors in a patient with dark teeth due to tetracycline staining.

enamel fractures away from the dentin (Fig. 4.41). Once the enamel fractures, the exposed dentin can be ground down rapidly, leaving only the roots. Radiographically, the enamel is barely visible and appears ghost-like or absent (Fig. 4.42). The treatment is to cap the teeth with full crowns or to extract the teeth and make dentures.

Dentinogenesis imperfecta (hereditary opalescent dentin) is more common than amelogenesis imperfecta and is characterized by irregular dentin formation in both the primary and permanent dentitions. It is a dominant inherited or sporadic genetic defect and is seen in 1 in 8000 individuals in the population. Clinically, the teeth are normal in contour on eruption. Characteristically, their color is blue, gray, or violet

and may have an opalescence (Fig. 4.43). The enamel chips away readily because of a defective dentinoenamel junction. This may lead to severe attrition similar to that seen in amelogenesis imperfecta. Radiographically, the characteristic changes noted are the obliteration of the pulp chamber, short roots, and constriction of the cementoenamel junction that gives the crown a bell-shaped appearance (Fig. 4.44). Dentinogenesis imperfecta is also seen in many cases of osteogenesis imperfecta, another hereditary disease characterized by imperfect formation of connective tissue resulting in fragile bone and blue sclerae of the eyes.

ACQUIRED TEETH DEFECTS

Certain defects of teeth are not developmental in the sense of being congenital. After the eruption of teeth, various factors

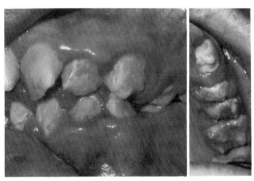

Figure 4.41. Amelogenesis imperfecta. All teeth were hypoplastic and hypocalcified. The enamel chips easily and is worn away. Other family members had a similar dentition. There are heavy calculus deposits on teeth.

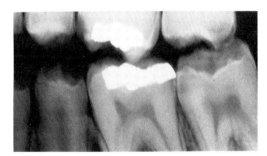

Figure 4.42. Amelogenesis imperfecta. Note absence and ghost-like appearance of enamel. All teeth are affected. Same patient as figure 4.41

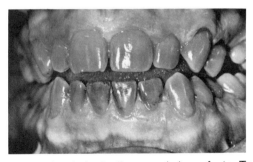

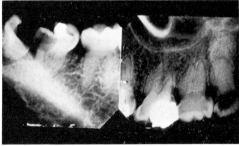

Figure 4.43. *Left*, dentinogenesis imperfecta. Teeth have gray color and opalescent hue. Patient's primary teeth were similarly affected. His mother had the same condition.
Figure 4.44. *Right*, radiographs of molar teeth of patient shown in Figure 4.43. Note bell-shaped crowns, constriction at the cementoenamel junction, lack of pulp chambers, sclerosed canals, and short roots. Patient presented with toothache due to extensive caries.

can exert themselves so that the teeth acquire characteristic lesions of the calcified surfaces. These are attrition, abrasion, and erosion.

Attrition is the normal wearing away of the biting surfaces of the teeth by mastication. This occurs in all individuals but may be more pronounced in some depending on personal habits and diet. The mamelons on newly erupted teeth are quickly worn away, except in individuals with an anterior open bite because the anterior teeth never meet. Some individuals clench and grind their teeth unconsciously and may speed the process of attrition. Rough, gritty food is another factor related to attrition. In severe cases the dentin is exposed, and in some instances the teeth appear to be cut in cross-section with a central darker area of secondary dentin appearing where the pulp originally was (Fig. 4.45). The dentin, when exposed, tends to stain brown by absorbing debris or tobacco stains. The worn surfaces are shiny and firm. In some cases, the pulp may become exposed. Pulpitis and periapical disease may then follow.

Abrasion is the pathologic wearing away of external tooth surfaces by mechanical means. Various abrasive agents may be responsible and can be determined usually by a careful history or astute observation. Because of the diversity of causes, the tooth defects will assume various shapes and forms. The surface of the defects are hard and smooth. Several examples will be noted. A patient with a full upper denture with porcelain teeth can wear away the natural teeth that remain in the lower jaw. Toothpicks, dental floss, bobbypins, nails, or any other item that is habitually and excessively used against the teeth will cause abrasion at the site of usage. Pipe smokers frequently hold the stem only in one position. After years, there is significant wearing and the teeth conform in shape to the pipestem (pipestem abrasion) (Fig. 4.46). Toothbrushing may cause abrasion at the cervical labial margins particularly if a back-and-forth motion is used. The resulting grooves in the cementum simulate erosion, but the defects are usually more severe on one side depending on the dexterity of the individual.

Erosion of teeth refers to the dissolution of the tooth by chemical means or by frictional intraoral forces not as yet defined. Characteristically erosive defects occur at the labial or buccal surfaces, particularly of the incisor teeth, at the cementoenamel junction; the biting surfaces are not involved. They appear as hard, smooth, shiny, ditch-like areas (Fig. 4.47). Other patterns of erosion may be seen such as on the lingual aspect or around the entire circumference of some teeth. Erosions are primarily idiopathic; however, some are associated with acids from foods, beverages, or gastric disturbances (Table 4.1). Patients who suck on lemons or drink large quantities of orange juice develop erosions on the

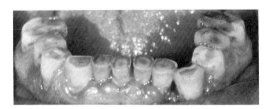

Figure 4.45. Severe attrition of mandibular teeth. The surfaces are flat, hard and shiny. Secondary dentin fills the pulp chamber area.

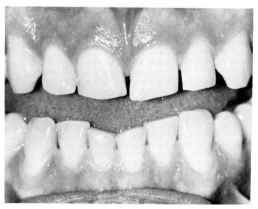

Figure 4.46. Pipestem abrasion of teeth. Pipestem has abraded mandibular central incisors.

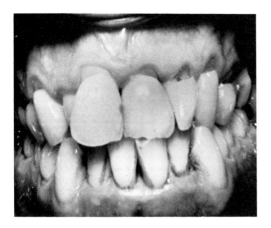

Figure 4.47. Dental erosion. Smooth, hard defects occurring at cervical margins of the teeth.

Table 4.1.
Causes of dental erosion

Dietary
  Fruits and food with citric acid
    Lemons, oranges, grapefruits, tomatoes,
      bananas
  Fruit juices
  Acid (carbonated) beverages
    Soft drinks; nondietetic and dietetic
  Vinegar—pickled foods
  Candy—sour balls, mints
  Cordials
  Vitamin C (chewable)
Medicinal
  HCl replacement
  Iron tonic
  Vitamin C
  Acid drops (tablets)
  Aspirin
Regurgitational
  Anorexia nervosa
  Vomiting
  Stress—reflux phenomenon
Occupational
  Industrial acids
  Gas chlorinated pools
Idiopathic
  Acid saliva

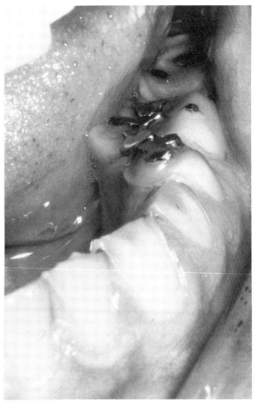

Figure 4.48. Severe dental erosion. Note the missing enamel and dentin and the fillings standing above the surface. The patient was diabetic and drank 15 sugar-free colas/day.

labial surfaces (Fig. 4.48). Erosive patterns can even be noted on restorations that are placed in teeth. Treatment is difficult because the erosion progresses even after the area is restored, although restorations do retard the process.

CHAPTER 5

Caries and Dental Pulp Disorders

DENTAL CARIES

Dental caries (tooth decay) is a progressive disease of the hard dental structures. It is characterized by decalcification, proteolysis, and microbial invasion and results in the destruction of the hard structures to form a cavity. It follows the interaction of three main factors, namely, the host (susceptible teeth), bacteria, and food (diet).

Dental caries is one of the most prevalent worldwide chronic diseases of man. Over 95% of the population have decay or will have had it before they die. Very few individuals are immune to it. However, current measures to control the disease especially through the use of systemic fluoride and topical applications are causing a decrease in occurrence.

Problems arise because of the complications stemming from decay. The hard dental structures are unique. Enamel is 97% mineralized (calcified). Dentin is about 70% mineralized and 30% of it is organic (cellular and pericellular material). Cementum is about 60% calcified. However, the teeth are not protected as are other systems by epithelium. Moreover, once the destructive process begins, it generally is progressive. Fluorides and remineralization procedures offer hope in controlling caries. The only means to date of repairing the destruction is by restorative dentistry, which is usually time-consuming and expensive. The challenge then is to overcome the complications of dental caries through prevention.

The etiology of dental caries in humans is still not settled. However, through laboratory and clinical research there is much that is known and certain generalizations can be made. Dental caries seems to be a multifactorial disease involving bacteria, food, and the tooth. It is an infectious disease because of the bacteria. These are endogenous bacteria that normally reside in the mouth. However, the bacteria involved differ for different sites of decay. In the pit and fissure lesions, nonspecific acid-producing bacteria are collected from the crevices. In smooth surface lesions, plaque-forming streptococci, *Streptococcus mutans*, are involved. They produce sticky substances, dextrans, which adhere to the teeth. In cemental or root surface lesions, the odontomyces viscosus organism is implicated.

The stagnation of food is related to decay. Food stagnates in pits and fissures (occlusal surfaces), beneath contact areas of teeth, at the cervical margins, beneath clasp arms of dentures, beneath overhanging margins on restorations, around orthodontic appliances, about crowded teeth, and in many other conditions. With the stagnation of food, bacteria can proliferate and yield metabolic products—some of which are acids. The acids are capable of demineralizing the tooth, and if the circumstances are proper (i.e. if the tooth is susceptible), the hard structure will begin to disintegrate and decay. Thus, there appear to be two processes, the production of the cariogenic agent (acid) and the production of a susceptible tooth surface on which the agent can act. A simplified schema for the pathogenesis of dental caries is:

$$food + bacteria \rightarrow acid$$

$$acid + tooth \rightarrow caries$$

There are many factors that alter or affect this process. The types of food most often incriminated are the carbohydrates, namely the sugars. Within 15 minutes after ingesting food, the acid content of the saliva rises to a level that can destroy tooth substance. This is particularly true for sweet foods. However, the length of time the food is present and the type of food are also factors. For instance, sticky foods such as toffee candy are more cariogenic than hard candy. But hard candy is usually held in the mouth for a long time. As long as it is there, the acid level will remain high. The frequency of eating is therefore important and in the snack-oriented United States will continue to be a major factor promoting caries. In the absence of refined carbohydrates there would be no decay, but it seems to be an unreasonable goal to remove them from the diet. Certainly, a moderate approach is recommended. In situations where a dietary history clearly defines this as a factor, then attempts at diminishing or substituting sugars are warranted.

Besides food there are other factors. Heredity may play a role, but it is not clearly defined because a true immunity to caries is rare. Interestingly, in the disease of mongolism, there is less evidence of decay, but more periodontal disorders. A study of the saliva from these patients has shown it to be less acidic than normal. Thus saliva may be a factor in caries. It is known that patients with a decrease in salivary flow or dry mouth (xerostomia) are more prone to decay.

Teeth are more prone to caries when they first appear in the mouth. This accounts for the fact that the decay rate is greatest during the years of eruption, falls after 25 years of age, and increases again in older age. The occlusal surface is the most susceptible to decay followed by the mesial,

distal, buccal, and lingual (except on the maxillary teeth where lingual surfaces decay more than buccal). The posterior teeth present more decay than the anterior teeth. The lower incisors appear to be the least susceptible but are usually involved in cases of severe or rampant caries. This order of susceptibility is a clinical fact and definitely relates to the order of eruption and the areas of stagnation that occur as the teeth erupt. The increase in decay in older age relates to the fact that more root surface is exposed as the gingiva recedes and the recession promotes the stagnation of food. Characteristically, the caries most prevalent in older age is cemental whereas the caries of youth is mostly pit and fissure and smooth surface.

The fluoride content of teeth affects the susceptibility to caries. If the fluoride content of drinking water is one part per million during the formation of the teeth, those teeth will be less susceptible to decay. Once the crown is calcified, systemic fluoride is of no benefit but topical application is, and remineralization of the outer surface may take place. Above one part per million, the teeth may develop fluorosis or mottled enamel. In this case there is still a reduction in decay despite the fact that there is hypocalcification and hypoplasia. Teeth with hypoplastic defects are not more prone to caries but can collect more debris which may promote the carious process.

Dental caries starts at the external surface of the tooth and progresses toward the pulp. The process in the enamel is mainly demineralization since the enamel is mostly calcified tissue. In the dentin demineralization, proteolysis (breakdown of the protein organic matter) and microbial invasion occurs. The pattern of decay can best be classified according to its clinical location, i.e. pit and fissure, smooth surface, and cemental caries (Fig. 5.1).

Pit and fissure caries is seen in areas normally considered self-cleansing. Food may stagnate in grooves and crevices of the occlusal surfaces of molars and premolars, buccal surfaces of mandibular molars, and

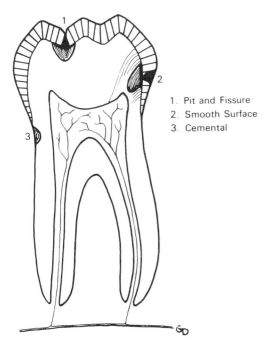

1. Pit and Fissure
2. Smooth Surface
3. Cemental

Figure 5.1. Dental caries. Patterns of dental caries in enamel and dentin according to surface involvement. *1*, pit and fissure caries; *2*, smooth surface caries; and *3*, cemental caries.

food debris that sticks to the tooth surface by gummy substances called dextrans. Streptococcal organisms are primarily responsible for producing these dextrans and for the production of the acids that can demineralize the tooth surface. The plaque covers a broad area and the carious lesion is therefore broader at the surface than pit and fissure lesions. The external surface outline is elliptical with the length of spread being in the buccolingual direction. In sections, the process follows the direction of the enamel rods in a triangular pattern with the base at the smooth surface and the apex toward the dentinoenamel junction. When the dentin is reached, there is lateral spread similar to that seen in the pit and fissure lesions. The decay involves more tubules and following the tubules spreads pulpally in a conical or triangular pattern with the apex toward the pulp (Fig. 5.2).

lingual surfaces of maxillary molar and anterior teeth. The pattern is one of a spreading cone following the enamel rods. In sections, the apex is at the occulusal surface and the base is toward the dentinoenamel junction. When the dentin is reached, there is a lateral spread along the dentinoenamel junction, undermining the enamel. As the process advances toward the pulp, it follows the course of the dentinal tubules in a conical pattern with its base at the dentinoenamel junction and its apex toward the pulp. Because of this pattern, the pit and fissure caries looks deceptively small at the surface. There may be only a pinpoint defect on exploration, but considerable other destruction must be assumed.

Smooth surface caries occurs in those areas of the tooth that are not self-cleaning. Usually this is at the interproximal area just below the contact point of adjacent teeth, where food debris stagnates. These areas are associated with plaque. Plaque is an invisible film of bacterial colonies and

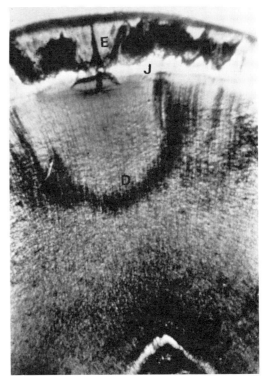

Figure 5.2. Ground section of tooth with smooth surface caries. Note *E*, multiple lesions in enamel; *J*, lateral spread along dentinoenamel junction; and *D*, pattern of decay in dentin, with apex toward the pulp.

As the caries progresses in the dentin, there are two protective mechanisms that can take place. The odontoblastic processes within the dentinal tubules degenerate, and the empty tubule becomes plugged with calcium salts and forms a harder or sclerotic dentin. This temporarily stops the advance of the process in those tubules. Unfortunately, the process can affect other tubules and continue toward the pulp (Fig. 5.3). Ultimately the calcified dentin is demineralized, bacteria invade the tubules, and the dentin decomposes and becomes softened.

The other protective mechanism is the formation of reparative or tertiary dentin. In the area of the pulp corresponding to the dentinal tubules involved with caries, the odontoblasts move toward the pulp and lay down new dentin behind them. This is to protect the pulp and reflects the fact that

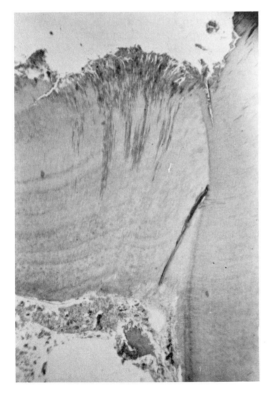

Figure 5.3. Decalcified section of molar tooth with extensive decay. Dark linear streaks represent bacterial colonies within dentinal tubules of reparative dentin. The pulp below is necrotic.

the best protection for the pulp is an adequate thickness of dentin. Therefore, early treatment of caries is essential in order to maintain this thickness of dentin.

Cemental caries, also called senile caries because of the general age of occurrence, presents a pattern similar to that of dentinal caries. Generally the enamel is not involved because of the recession of the gingiva. The caries starts at Sharpey's fibers (a type of collagen fiber in the cementum) and spreads rapidly in a broad outline. In sections, the spread is more apical but follows the dentinal tubules in a triangular pattern with the apex toward the pulp. Clinically there may be only a small opening but the lesion may be quite advanced.

Clinically, the naked eye cannot detect the initiation of the carious lesion (Fig. 5.4). As decalcification occurs the enamel may appear as chalky white. With an explorer this may feel smooth so that cavitation is no criterion for judging the extent of the lesion. With time cavitation may occur and bacteria penetrating the cavity and dentin will cause a brown stain (Fig. 5.5). Because of the undermining of the enamel, it may fracture easily. The demineralization dentin may be softened and easily removed with an excavator.

The dental radiograph is an adjunct in determining caries, particularly interproximal lesions. On the radiograph, the hard tooth structure appears gray-white and is radiopaque. The pulp stops less x-rays, appears dark, and is radiolucent. Dental caries is seen as a radiolucent lesion; the pattern mimics that previously described (Fig. 5.1) (Figs. 5.6 and 5.7). The radiograph, however, is merely a shadow. In fact, the carious process on a radiograph usually underestimates the actual extent of involvement (Fig. 5.4). Despite this caution, the radiograph is most useful in detecting interproximal caries which clinically may be undetected by explorer because of lack of a rough enamel surface or cemental caries hidden beneath the gingiva.

Usually there are no symptoms of dental caries. There may be slight pain stimulated by heat, cold, or sweets that disappears

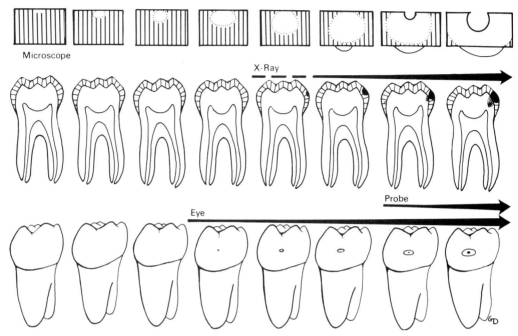

Figure 5.4. Schematic diagram tracing the progression of dental caries on the distal aspect of a mandibular molar. *Top* line indicates microscopic appearance in enamel (*vertical lines*) and then dentin. Lesion starts at surface long before it can be detected by *eye, x-ray*, or *probe. Middle* drawings depict cross-section in mesiodistal dimension. *Bottom* drawings depict distal view of tooth. Once decalcification is well established in enamel, the eye can detect a white lesion clinically. The x-ray is not as sensitive as the eye but is essential for proximal lesions. The probe can palpate a lesion only when a cavitation or surface breakdown has occurred.

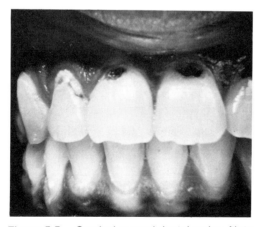

Figure 5.5. Cervical enamel dental caries. Note progression from left to right to opaque lesion to cavitation with deep staining. An earlier opaque lesion appears on the cervical third of the mandibular cuspid.

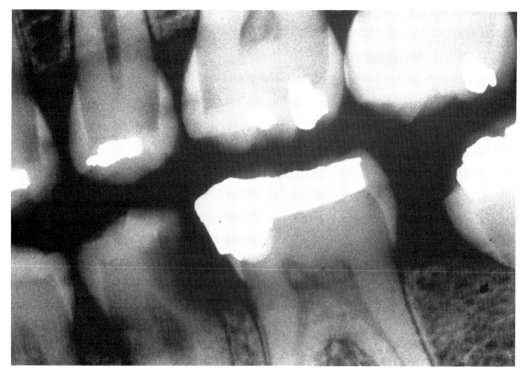

Figure 5.6.   Bitewing radiograph showing multiple smooth surface carious lesions.

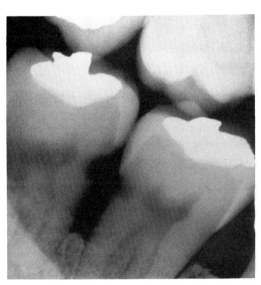

Figure 5.7. Bitewing radiograph showing cemental caries of second and third mandibular molars.

when the stimulus is removed. But most often caries is progressive, yet symptomless.

Although most decay is chronic and progressive, there are two other types recognized in terms of activity, these being considered extremes of the basic chronic type. One is acute caries which, as the term implies, runs a rapid and painful course. There usually is no defensive activity and the pulp is quickly involved. The other type is arrested caries and indicates that the process is in a state of inactivity. Arrested decay is seen commonly in children with large occlusal lesions in which the decayed surface becomes essentially open and self-cleansing. In these instances the decayed dentin wears away and leaves a hard, brown-stained remineralized dentin. The same phenomenon is seen on proximal surfaces with caries exposed after the extraction of an adjacent tooth or on cervical or cemental caries exposed after recession of the gingiva (Fig. 5.8).

The treatment for dental caries is restorative dentistry, utilizing various restorative materials to replace the destroyed tooth

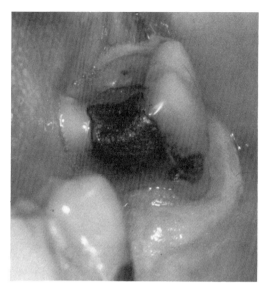

Figure 5.8. Arrested dental caries on exposed mesial root surface of mandibular molar. It is firm and very blackened.

substance. Because of the magnitude of problems, the dental profession is endeavoring to control and prevent dental caries by various means, including the use of fluorides and bonding agents.

PULPITIS

Pulpitis refers to inflammation of the pulp. The dental pulp is a loose cellular connective tissue with branching and anastomosing neurovascular channels. Pulp is unique in that it is surrounded by rigid dentin, and it has no collateral circulation because the dental arteries are end arteries. Specialized cells of the pulp are the odontoblasts which line the outer layer of the pulp and communicate to the dentinoenamel junction by long extensions of their cell bodies lying within the dentinal tubules. These cells are responsible for the sensitivity of teeth and for the formation of secondary or reparative dentin. Despite these unique features, inflammation of the pulp is like inflammation of connective tissue anywhere else in the body.

Pulpitis is somewhat difficult to understand because the clinical symptoms and signs that occur cannot be correlated to changes which occur histologically. Therefore, it will be discussed in relation to the various pulpal irritants and the possible pulpal responses that can occur. In general, the effect of the irritant is balanced by the resistance of the host. If the resistance is low, the result may be severe with necrosis of the pulp. Conversely, the irritant may be severe but the pulpal response may be limited and quite favorable. In this circumstance, the damage to the pulp may be reversible and the pulp can be repaired. Yet, such severe damage may cause irreversible damage and may lead to further consequences.

The pulpal irritants are microorganisms, traumatic, iatrogenic, chemical, idiopathic, and systemic.

The most common cause of pulpitis is microbial with the bacteria of dental caries being primarily responsible. Bacterial toxins, bacteria themselves, or products of degradation caused by their invasion can cause inflammation.

Other avenues for bacteria are dental erosion, attrition, fractures of teeth, and periodontal disease. Pulps may be affected in periodontal disease via lateral canals and via the apical foramen in cases of severe disease.

Trauma from fractures, blows, or bruxing (grinding) of the teeth can irritate the pulp.

Iatrogenic causes are those that are introduced by the person performing a treatment or service. Simply preparing a tooth for a restoration has an effect on the pulp. In this regard, a high speed water-cooled drill with light pressure is least damaging to the pulp. Even polishing of the teeth can cause pulpitis. The rubber polishing cup is capable of generating sufficient heat to cause thermal changes that affect pulpal tissue via the odontoblasts. Restorations that replaced destroyed tooth structures can cause similar changes. Amalgam and gold respond to thermal changes differently than dentin.

Chemicals cause pulpal changes. Various chemicals are applied to the dentinal tubules in the form of fillings, bases, and disinfectants. Unlined composite restorations may cause low grade chronic pulpitis. The eugenol in the temporary dressing, zinc oxide and eugenol, is used to relieve the pain of toothache but is also a pulpal irritant.

Idiopathic causes are unknown or vague. Most pulpal disorders occur in or are associated with older pulps. Thus aging appears to be a factor. An older pulp has less cells and more fibrous tissue so that resistance may be lowered with age because there are less cell available to respond favorably. Resorptions of the dentin are other causes that can be listed as idiopathic.

Systemic causes reflect the fact that the pulp is not divorced from the general circulation. For example, diabetic patients are prone to bacterial infections. These patients commonly have multiple infected pulps. In patients with sickle cell anemia, with less oxygen available, there may be a pulpitis without caries or other irritants.

No matter what the irritant is, the pulp can respond basically in only two ways: clinically and histologically. There may be pain, no pain, reparative dentin formation, or a spectrum of inflammatory changes.

Eighty percent of toothaches are due to pulpitis or pulp-related periapical inflammation. Pain, then, is a major pulpal response. Pain results from the increase of pressure within the confined pulp and from the shifting of the fluid medium of the pulp. The stimulus for pain can be heat, cold, sweets, air, or inflammatory exudation. Regardless of the stimulus, the result will be pain and this can be categorized in terms of duration, frequency, intensity, and character.

Pulpalgia refers to pain in the pulp. Generally speaking, pain of short duration that disappears on removal of a stimulus is favorable. That which lingers is unfavorable for the vitality of the pulp. Previous episodes of pain in a tooth (frequency) are also a sign of pulpal destruction and irreversibility. The pain may be acute, being of short

duration but severe. This type is associated with pulp abscesses and pulps with partial necrosis, is usually well localized, and the tooth may be sensitive to percussion (tapping or biting). Chronic pain, on the other hand, is usually vague and intermittent.

When a toothache occurs, one usually finds a carious tooth, a lost restoration, or a chipped tooth. Other pains mistaken for toothaches are the result of dental erosion or periodontal inflammation—usually due to food impaction and maxillary sinusitis. Another aspect to be considered is referred pain. For instance, a pulpitis in a lower right second premolar may refer pain to the right ear and the right temple.

There may be no clinical manifestations of pulpitis. That is, there can be pulpitis without pain. Clinically, painless pulpitis can be suspected. A tooth with an existing deep restoration of amalgam or a full crown probably has some pulpitis although there may be no history of pain.

Histologically, there are several possible responses. The most favorable response is the formation of reparative dentin. This occurs in the advance of dental caries and also in response to the preparation of teeth for restoration. So long as there are healthy odontoblasts, there can be dentin formation, the mechanism of the tooth to insulate the pulp from an irritant. If there is at least 1 mm of remaining dentin, the pulpal damage will be minimal.

In histologic pulpitis, the connective tissue is usually involved with a chronic inflammatory response. Assuming an irritant, the first change is the degeneration and necrosis of odontoblasts. As these die, there is undoubtedly an initial acute inflammatory response, but the typical neutrophilic response is rarely seen on microscopic sections. What is seen is a condition called hyperemia which refers to blood vessels congested with red blood cells, but none of the red blood cells are seen outside the vessels. This may be the first sign of inflammation in the pulp. With time chronic cells and fluid appear. The pulp can repair by forming new odontoblasts to lay down dentin, or it may remain in a state of chronic inflammation (Fig. 5.9). This may be confined to the coronal portion or, depending on resistance, may involve all of the pulp. If the pulp does not repair, and this can include the formation of dense connective tissue, it may undergo necrosis and death. In some pulps, a whole spectrum of inflammatory events can be seen. Clinically, it is a challenge to guess at the histologic state of the pulp.

In a carious tooth in particular, there may be a pulpal abscess. One or more abscesses can occur in the pulp horn. As more and more bacteria or toxins invade the pulp, neutrophils try to engulf them. A collection of neutrophils, dead and dying, plus bacteria in a liquid state, forms and becomes encapsulated. This is a pulpal abscess and is associated with severe pain (Fig. 5.10). Most often there is normal pulp tissue below the abscess so that if the abscess or pus is removed for treatment (pulpotomy) the pulp would likely heal. However, clinically one can only guess at the possibility of an abscess being present. A decision that there is irreversible pulpitis is followed by endodontic therapy.

Chronic hyperplastic pulpitis (pulp polyp) is a dramatic and relatively frequent type of pulpal response. It is seen in younger pulps, mainly children and young adults, of primary molars and first and

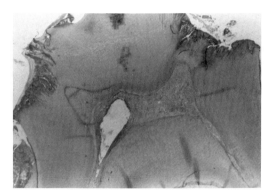

Figure 5.10. A pulpal abscess in decalcified tooth with extensive dentinal caries and reparative dentin of pulp horns. The cleared area in vivo was filled with liquified necrotic pulp and neutrophils.

second permanent molars. Generally, the decay rate has been sufficiently rapid so that the crown disintegrates and the pulp becomes exposed. The pulp responds with chronic inflammation in the coronal pulp. However, there is a build up of granulation tissue (hyperplasia), and with time this type of tissue grows toward the open space. It looks like a grape or polyp extending from the pulp (Fig. 5.11). It usually fills the defect of the crown and often mimics hyperplastic gingivae. Because of the new blood vessels in granulation tissue, the pulp polyp is a red-pink and tends to bleed readily when probed. However, there is no sensitivity because granulation tissue contains no nerve tissue. The underlying pulpal tissue often is intact and uninflamed, a sign of excellent host resistance. Therefore, the pulp polyp can be treated by pulpotomy if the tooth is restorable. Otherwise root canal therapy or extraction must be done.

The complication of pulpitis is that the inflammation will progress beyond the root apex into the periapical area. The sequelae of pulpitis are the dentoalveolar abscess, cellulitis, periapical granuloma, or cyst.

The treatment of pulpitis depends on the determination based on clinical signs and symptoms as to whether the damage is reversible or irreversible (ultimately leading to pulpal necrosis). There is no reliable

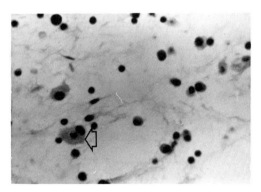

Figure 5.9. Chronic inflammatory cells. Lymphocytes, plasma cells, macrophages. Macrophage with phagocytized cell (*arrow*).

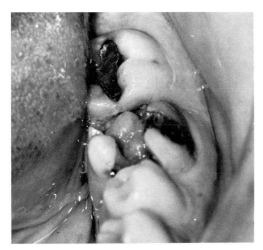

Figure 5.11. Pulp polyp. Inflamed tissue from pulp extends to fill space of crown lost by rapid decay.

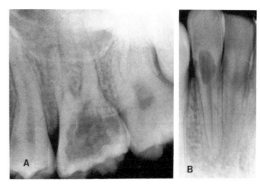

Figure 5.12. *A,* internal resorption of maxillary molar crown. The external surface of the tooth appeared normal but was pink. *B,* internal resorption of mandibular incisor. The pulp area is expanded.

means of determining the vitality of the pulp. Pulp testers, thermal responses, are merely aids and in no way indicate actual vitality. Radiographically, there are no discernible changes. For reversible pulpitis the treatment is a pulpal dressing and new restoration of pulpotomy. For irreversible pulpitis, pulpectomy and root canal therapy or extraction is required.

Internal resorption or idiopathic resorption refers to the destruction of the dentin from the pulpal side toward the outside of the tooth. The cause is unknown; however, a history of trauma may be elicited. The dentin is whittled away by giant cells, and this process may continue rapidly or stop spontaneously. Internal resorption is asymptomatic and is noted on routine radiographs as ballooning radiolucent expansion of the pulp usually in the root (Fig. 5.12). It may occur in the pulp of the crown in which case the pink tissue of the pulp shows through the enamel (pink tooth). The treatment is root canal therapy. If the resorption perforates the periodontal ligament, the tooth is treated by extraction.

External resorption of teeth is more common than internal resorption. It occurs naturally in the shedding of primary teeth and microscopically on most teeth. Occasion-

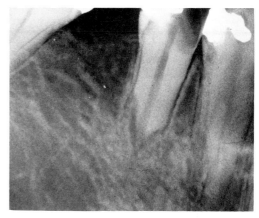

Figure 5.13. External resorption of root. Note irregular outline of apical end of root.

ally, however, it is progressive. External resorption refers to the loss of cementum and dentin of a tooth from the external surface in toward the pulp. Radiographically it is seen as an irregular loss of root structures (Fig. 5.13). Known causes are periapical inflammation, reimplantation of teeth, tumors and cysts, excessive forces (orthodontic), impacted teeth, and idiopathic forces (Fig. 5.14). The treatment is to diagnose the cause and to remove it. The resorbed portion of the root will not heal but will not progress further after therapy.

Pulp stones are gross calcifications occurring in the pulp (Fig. 5.15). They are very common. Radiographically, they appear as small, rounded radiopaque (white) masses within the pulp chamber or canal (Fig. 5.14). The cause is unknown. They are also referred to as denticles because some of them are composed of dentin. They do not cause pain and may interfere with root canal therapy.

SEQUELAE OF PULPITIS

The extension of inflammation of the pulp beyond the tooth into the periodontal ligament area represents periapical inflammation. In many instances the pulp is necrotic. However, periapical inflammation can be present despite vital tissue being in the pulp. There are three common lesions that may follow pulpitis, namely the periapical abscess, granuloma, and cyst (Table 5.1).

The periapical or dentoalveolar abscess is an acute or chronic suppurative (pus-producing) process in the periapices or radicular area of the involved tooth. The usual cause is untreated dental caries, but a periodontal pocket or a partially erupted

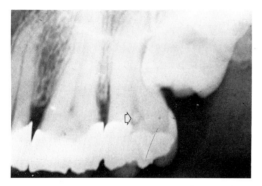

Figure 5.14. External resorption of root of second molar by pressure from impacted third molar. Also note opaque object within pulp chamber of second molar (pulp stone, *arrow*).

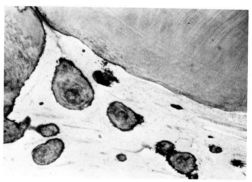

Figure 5.15. Numerous pulp stones within pulp of a tooth.

Table 5.1.
Periapical sequelae of pulpitis

	Abscess	Granuloma	Cyst

Clinical	Acute:
	  Severe pain
	  Extrusion
	  Parulis
	  Cellulitis
	Chronic
	  no pain
	  fistula
		Little or none	None

Radiographic	Early: none Late: radiolucent	Radiolucent	Radiolucent

Microscopic	Acute:
	  Pus
	Chronic:
	  Pus
	  Granuloma or Cyst
		Chronic Inflammation
		Granulation tissue
		Fibrosis
			Lumen
			Epithelial lining
			Chronic inflammation
			Fibrotic wall

Treatment	1. Drain pus 2. Root canal or 3. Extraction	1. Root canal, or 2. Apicoectomy or 3. Extraction	1. Root canal 2. Apicoectomy, or 3. Extraction

third molar may be other etiologic factors. Clinically, acute periapical abscesses are responsible for severe pain. The build-up of pus and edema at the root end causes pressure which acts on nerve endings in the periodontal ligament and elicits pain. In addition the inflammatory exudate pushes against the root causing the tooth to extrude. The affected tooth then touches its opponent first and causes more pain. Diagnostically the tooth is sensitive to percussion so that tapping teeth can locate the offending tooth. If the abscess forms immediately following the extension of inflammation into the periapical region, there may be no indication on a radiograph of periapical destruction. In these acute abscesses there may be only a slight widening of the periodontal ligament at the tooth apex (Figs. 5.16 and 5.17). If, on the other hand, the abscess originates in a preexisting granuloma or cyst, there will be a clearly defined radiolucent shadow about the root or beyond it, corresponding to the destruction of the granuloma or cyst. The pain, however, will be a manifestation of the abscess.

The nature of pus within tissue is to find an exit or drainage. Consequently, the treatment is to establish drainage. This is done by opening directly into the pulp chamber of the tooth or by extraction. The pressure of the suppurative process is released and, dramatically, the pain is abated. Patients may have additional symptoms of fever and malaise which should be treated on an individual basis. Often antibiotics are necessary.

If the tooth is not drained or removed, the natural course of the periapical abscess proceeds to establish drainage. The pus burrows through the alveolar bone forming a channel called a sinus or a fistula that eventually open to an outer surface. Generally, it follows a pathway of least resistance. After exiting the bone to the buccal or labial, lingual or palate, the suppuration may form a painful, red swelling beneath the mucosa called a gumboil or parulis (Fig. 5.18). A gumboil (suppurative, painful

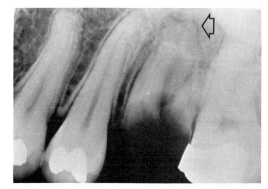
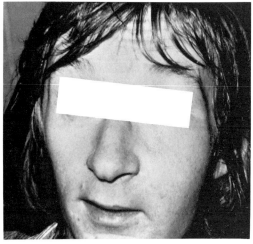

Figure 5.16. Acute dentoalveolar abscess, maxillary first molar. Note retained roots after loss of crown due to caries. Note widened periodontal membrane and loss of lamina dura at apices of roots (*arrow*).

Figure 5.17. Acute dentoalveolar abscess. Same patient as in Figure 5.16. Note swelling obliterating nasolabial fold, causing left eye to close.

swelling of the gingiva) may result from periodontal disease or foreign implanted material as well. Ultimately the gingival or palatal abscess may drain spontaneously (Fig. 5.19). Clinically, this mucosal abscess may be drained by incision and drainage often by starting the endodontic therapy. Upon drainage, the pain subsides. The patient may give a history of foul taste and no swelling or pain for a chronic dentoalveolar abscess. With spontaneous drainage, there remains a small red pimple-like lesion with a central fistulous opening. The fistula

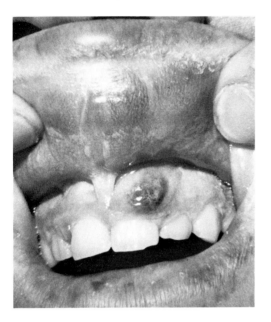

Figure 5.18. Gingival abscess or gumboil representing exit of inflammation originating at apices of maxillary left central incisor. Patient's lip was swollen with a cellulitis.

then connects the mucosa with the destruction at the end of the involved tooth (Figs. 5.20 and 5.21). This tract heals after treatment.

The pus may, in some instances, burrow through the bone deeper than alveolar bone and exit in areas other than mucosal surfaces. It can follow along sheaths of connective tissue that outline muscle and through the muscle itself. For instance, a lower molar may drain above the mylohyoid muscle of the floor of the mouth and present as a gingival abscess. But if it drains below the mylohyoid, a large hard swelling of the lower face may occur. This represents the spread of inflammation along the muscle and is termed cellulitis. It may be seen with or without a parulis being present. Patients with cellulitis are quite sick with fever and pain. The process may continue with spontaneous drainage onto the face thus forming an oral-facial or oral cutaneous fistula (Fig. 5.22). Excluding trauma, the periapical or dentoalveolar abscess is the most common cause of facial swelling.

The periapical or dental granuloma is one of the most common lesions seen in a dental office. It represents long-standing inflammation in the bone at the root end of the tooth. There usually is no clinical sign or symptom. The tooth may have had a prior history of pain or some slight sensitivity. Vitality testing usually indicates necrosis of the pulp. With the extension of inflammation into the radicular alveolar bone, a chronic inflammation is set up and persists. With time the periodontal ligament is destroyed and the bone is invaded by the extension of inflammatory cells. The process smolders without symptoms. Granulation tissue plus fibrous tissue replace the bone and its marrow. Often, giant cells, cholesterol and foam cells, all chronic cells indicating long-standing inflammation, are also seen. The process usually becomes self-limiting but never heals and a circumscribed area of granulating tissue (thus, granuloma) remains until treatment is instituted. On a radiograph, the granuloma appears as a radiolucency, usually clearly demarcated, about the apical portion of the involved tooth (Figs. 5.23 and 5.24). Treatment consists of root canal therapy or extraction. After therapy the localized area of destruction heals and new bone forms to obliterate the defect on a radiograph.

The periapical or radicular (root end) cyst is as common as the dental granuloma from which it is derived. Clinically, these

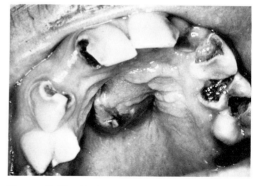

Figure 5.19. Palatal abscess with some drainage. Note many carious teeth which also had periapical involvement.

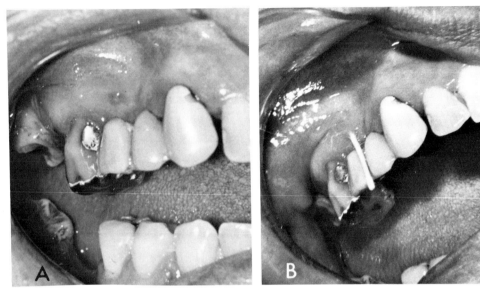

Figure 5.20. *A*, fistula on alveolar mucosa above second bicuspid pontic area of bridge in a patient with a chronic dentoalveolar abscess. and no pain, but foul taste. *B*, gutta percha point inserted into fistulous opening, without anesthesia.

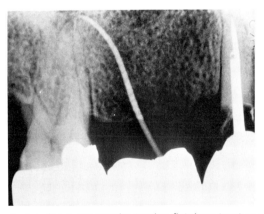

Figure 5.21. Radiograph showing gutta percha tracing fistulous tract or sinus which extended from the first molar tooth (same patient as shown in Figure 5.20).

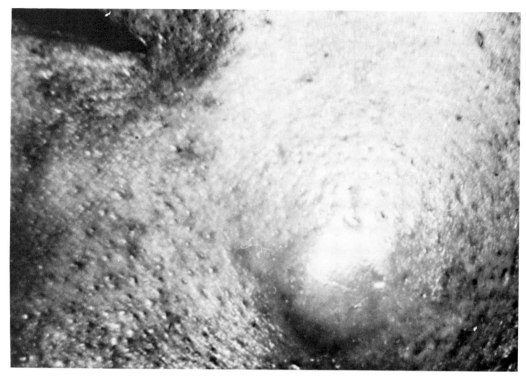

Figure 5.22. Facial abscess near corner of mouth about to drain or be drained. This abscess generated from an abscessed tooth.

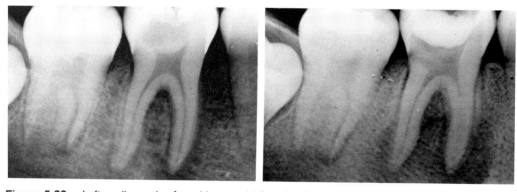

Figure 5.23. *Left*, radiograph of an 11-year-old female. First molar has extensive occlusal caries, periapical inflammation of both roots.
Figure 5.24. *Right*, radiograph of same patient as in Figure 5.23, 6 months later showing progressive involvement of bone and enlarged and more prominent radiolucencies about the roots. The lesion was a dental granuloma with abscess and the patient had an enlarged jaw (see Fig. 5.30).

cysts are asymptomatic. The involved teeth are usually necrotic. Radiographically, the radicular cyst resembles the dental granuloma and chronic abscess with an area of radiolucent bone loss (Fig. 5.25). The radiograph cannot be used to distinguish the nature of the lesion. (A radiograph merely shows shadows, which is not a diagnosis.

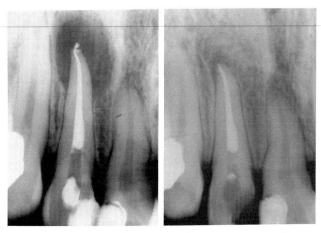

Figure 5.25. Periapical inflammatory lesion, a granuloma, or cyst or abscess. Sequential photos show *left*, root canal therapy completed and *right*, subsequent healing of periapical area by regeneration of bone.

Therefore, a periapical radiolucency is consistent most often with a granuloma, a cyst, or an abscess). The cyst is diagnosed because of its microscopic features.

By definition a cyst is a sac of fibrous tissue containing fluid or semisolid material, like cells, in a lumen which is lined by epithelium. The radicular cyst is derived from the epithelial rests of Malassez which are within the periodontal membrane surrounding a tooth (Fig. 5.26). In the presence of chronic inflammation of the granuloma, the epithelial rests proliferate (Fig. 5.27). Sometimes, the growing ball of epithelial cells enlarges to such a degree that the

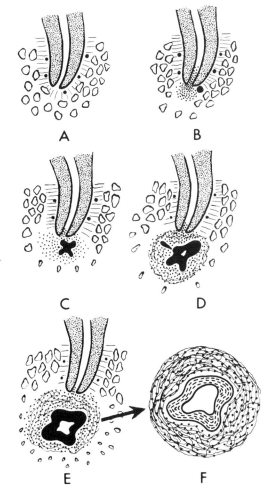

Figure 5.26. Schematic diagram depicting the development of a periapical cyst. *A*, normal root apex with adjacent periodontal ligament containing epithelial rests of Malassez (*black dots*), and clear areas surrounding root represent alveolar bone; *B*, inflammation from pulp extends into periapical area (granuloma) where bone is resorbed, and epithelial rest near the inflammation has begun to proliferate and is larger; *C*, continued growth of granuloma and rest epithelium; *D*, early liquefaction necrosis in center of epithelial mass; *E*, cyst with central lumen; and *F*, expanded view, lumen in center has fluid, surrounded by stratified squamous epithelium which is contained within connective tissue that is inflamed.

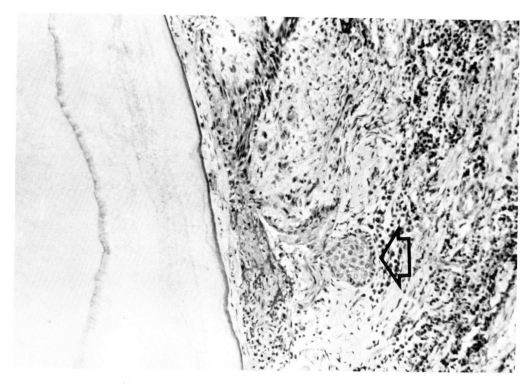

Figure 5.27.   Proliferating epithelium (*arrow*) within granuloma at root end of tooth (*left*).

nutrients to the central core of cells is too far removed from the connective tissue that contains the blood supply. Those central cells undergo necrosis and liquefy (liquefaction necrosis). This forms a small cavity or lumen with fluid and/or cells lined by epithelium (cyst). This inflammatory cyst can continue to enlarge and replace the apical alveolar bone. They may become several centimeters in size (Figs. 5.28 and 5.29). Following treatment the bone usually regenerates. Sometimes it may not and scar tissue repair persists (apical scar), leaving a radiolucent, asymptomatic lesion that does not enlarge. Both the cystic cavity and the cyst wall account for the cystic cavity and the cyst wall account for the radiolucent radiographic appearance. The treatment for radicular cyst is root canal therapy or extraction and surgical removal of the cyst.

Besides the periapical granuloma, cyst and abscess, there are other sequelae to pulpitis. There may be an infection of the

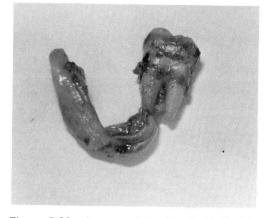

Figure 5.28.   Large periapical cyst attached to the root of a molar. The sac was originally filled with fluid. The bone defect extended from second molar to first bicuspid.

jaw bone, osteomyelitis, caused by various organisms. It is characterized by pain and sometimes by the death of the bone (a sequestrum) which must be removed. Two that are exaggerated spread of the inflam-

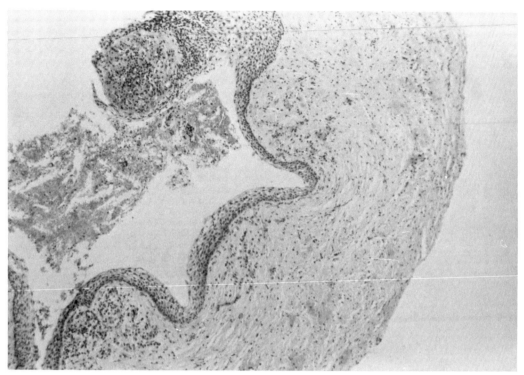

Figure 5.29. Cyst wall. Lumen (*left*) with fluid and debris, epithelial lining, and connective tissue wall.

mation are Ludwig's angina and cavernous sinus thrombosis. Though both are rare, they are life threatening. Ludwig's angina is a painful purulent inflammation spreading in the submandibular spaces and ultimately the pharynx that can choke the patient. In cavernous sinus thrombosis, the inflammation spreads rapidly from the face to the brain and a thrombus affects vital parts. Infections other than from pulpitis may cause these. Both conditions require hospitalization and high dosages of antibiotics.

Two other sequelae are characterized by the proliferation of bone. In Garré's osteomyelitis, there usually is a painful swelling of the mandible similar to a cellulitis and secondary to an infected radicular granuloma or cyst. But the swelling is firm because there is extra bone formed on the outer (periosteal) surface of the mandible (Fig. 5.30). After the tooth is treated by

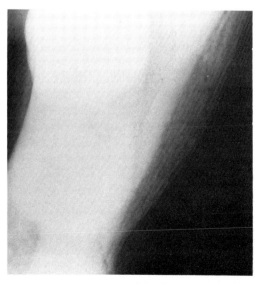

Figure 5.30. Proliferation of periosteal bone causing swelling of mandible in a young patient with an abscessed tooth (Garré's osteomyelitis).

endodontics or extraction, the bone remodels and the swelling subsides.

Condensing osteitis (focal sclerosing osteitis) is a common sequela to low grade pulpitis. It is usually seen as a radiopaque lesion associated with the roots of the mandibular molar teeth, usually the mesial root of the first molar. It occurs in younger people on a tooth with caries or a large restoration. Instead of the apical bone resorbing, the low grade inflammation induces extra dense bone to form. There is mild inflammation. Unless the tooth is symptomatic, no treatment is required. In theory, the opacity should decrease after endodontic therapy. However, it may persist in the bone after extraction of the tooth; then it is called a bone scar, an area of osteosclerosis.

Cysts other than radicular cysts do occur in the head and neck but their frequency is far less than the radicular cyst. Like the radicular cyst, the cyst is an abnormal sac or fibrous tissue, containing fluid or cells or more solid material. Lining the lumen is epithelium from which the cyst was derived. Unlike the radicular cyst, the cause for the development of the other cysts is unknown. Epithelial remnants or rests proliferate but not due to inflammation. Thus there may be no inflammation associated with these other cysts unless there is secondary infection or irritation. In other words, they are noninflammatory cysts. They are expansile, usually asymptomatic, lesions occurring in soft tissue but mostly bone. In either case they may be discovered routinely by noticing a swelling or a radiolucent area on radiographs. The area of destruction is always greater than that outlined on the radiograph. The radiographic appearance and site may suggest the presence of a cyst. However, cysts, abscesses, benign and malignant neoplasms, metabolic diseases, trauma, surgically removed tissue, and normal structures can all produce radiolucent areas on radiographs. Therefore, the final diagnosis can be made only after considering the radiographic image, an adequate history, other clinical features, and microscopic analysis.

Cysts are derived from embryonic epithelium that in development remains as a small cluster of cells entrapped in bone or soft tissue. For convenience cysts are classified as odontogenic, if they are derived from epithelium related to tooth development, or nonodontogenic. The following classification is offered with additional comments relevant to frequency and location of developmental cysts of the head and neck (Table 5.2) (Fig. 5.31).

Periodontal cysts arise from the epithelial rests of Malassez remaining in the periodontal ligament. The periapical cyst is the most common of all the cysts and has been covered in detail. It occurs in both the maxilla and mandible in relation to inflammation proceeding from the pulp. The residual cyst is a periapical cyst that persists after the removal of the involved tooth. The cyst is not curetted effectively at surgery, fails to heal, and remains (Fig. 5.32). The

Table 5.2.
Developmental cysts

I. Odontogenic: dental origin
  A. Periodontal: rests of Malassez in periodontal ligament
    1. Periapical: most common
    2. Residual: no tooth present
    3. Lateral periodontal
  B. Follicular: dental lamina, dental follicle, enamel organ
    1. Primordial: no tooth present
    2. Dentigerous: common
    3. Eruption
    4. Gingival: soft tissue
  C. Globulomaxillary: between lateral and canine
  D. Odontogenic keratocyst: recurrence
II. Nonodontogenic: Nondental origin
  A. Bony (fissural): rests in areas of fusion of developing processes
    1. Nasoplatine (incisive canal): common; midline
    2. Median palatine: midline
    3. Median mandibular: very rare
  B. Soft tissue
    1. Nasolabial (nasoalveolar)
    2. Lymphoepithelial
      Lateral neck (branchial cleft)
      Floor of mouth, etc.: oral tonsils
    3. Dermoid: floor, mouth, neck; midline
    4. Thyroglossal duct: midline

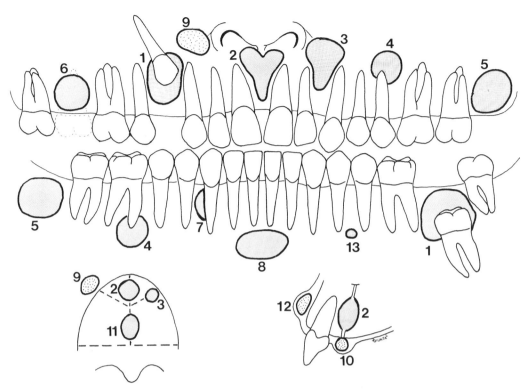

Figure 5.31. Various developmental cysts. Shaded cysts would be radiolucencies within bone. Stippled cysts would be in soft tissue, causing no radiolucency unless there is pressure atrophy of bone. *1*, dentigerous; *2*, nasopalatine (incisive canal); *3*, globulomaxillary; *4*, periapical (radicular); *5*, primordial, *6*, residual; *7*, lateral periodontal; *8*, median mandibular; *9*, nasolabial (nasoalveolar); *10*, incisive papillary; *11*, median palatal; *12*, gingival; and *13*, mental foramen (not a cyst). The odontogenic keratocyst has specific histology and radiographically could appear like *1*, *3*, *5*, *7*, or even *4*.

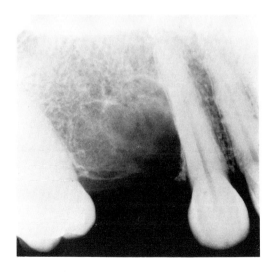

Figure 5.32. Residual cyst. This represents a periapical cyst which surrounded a tooth that was extracted.

lateral periodontal cyst occurs at the middle third of the root of a tooth that usually tests vital. This cyst is associated with periodontal disease or trauma.

The follicular cysts arise from epithelium associated with tooth development. The primordial cyst arises from a tooth germ that fails to form. Therefore, there is a history of a missing tooth, most commonly the mandibular third molar. This cyst must be distinguished from the residual cyst by an accurate history. The dentigerous cyst is the most common follicular cyst (Fig. 5.33). It is always associated with a tooth which is part of the wall of the cyst. It occurs particularly about impacted mandibular third molars and maxillary cuspids and is responsible for considerable bone destruction and possible swelling (Fig.

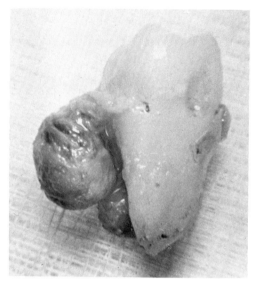

Figure 5.33. Dentigerous cyst or lateral periodontal cyst. Saclike structure contained fluid.

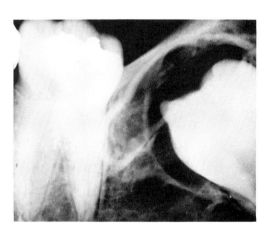

Figure 5.34. Radiolucency about crown of impacted third molar. Consistent with dentigerous cyst.

neously, with further eruption of the tooth into the oral cavity, or it may be surgically removed. The gingival cyst is derived from epithelium of the dental lamina and there are two types, both in soft tissue. Gingival cysts of the newborn (Epstein's pearls) occur in most infants. They are pearl-like keratin-filled cysts on the gum pads. They disappear quickly and spontaneously as the cysts open into the oral cavity.

The gingival cyst of the adult is rare. The counterpart of the lateral periodontal cyst, it occurs labially on the attached or unattached gingiva and appears similar to a mucocele. With pressure atrophy of the bone, there can be a radiolucency. Treatment is surgical removal.

The globulomaxillary cyst, in the past considered to be a fissural cyst, is probably a lateral periodontal cyst, a primordial, or a lateral dentigerous cyst derived from the respective odontogenic epithelium. It is characterized by its specific location, between the maxillary lateral and canine teeth. Usually it appears as an inverted pear-shaped radiolucency causing divergence of those roots. The teeth are usually vital although a radicular granuloma or cyst of either tooth could look similar radiographically. Treatment is surgical enucleation.

5.34). Rarely, tumors, such as ameloblastoma or carcinoma, may arise in the wall of a dentigerous cyst. Moreover, there are several odontogenic tumors that can have the same radiographic pattern as a dentigerous cyst. The eruption cyst occurs over erupting teeth and thus is seen mainly in children. It is seen clinically as a blue-purple mucosal swelling over the erupting tooth and resembles a blood blister (Fig. 5.35). The cyst usually disappears sponta-

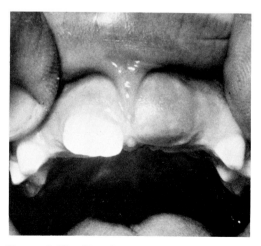

Figure 5.35. Eruption cyst overlying erupting left maxillary central incisor. Mucosa was bluish-purple in color.

The odontogenic keratocyst, derived most likely from dental lamina, is an unusual cyst that has an aggressive behavior in that it can recur following surgical excision. The name is derived from the histologic pattern which is specific and unique. One of the features is keratin formation. They may appear in several locations, commonly the posterior mandible in the form of a primordial cyst. Many of the other odontogenic cysts already covered may be a keratocyst. Because of their behavior they are called by their histologic name rather than the location in the jaw. They may cause extensive bone destruction and may recur several times. Rarely, they occur in patients with the basal cell nevus syndrome.

The nonodontogenic include the fissural cysts and other cysts that occur in specific locations in soft tissue. The fissural cysts are developmental occuring from epithelial remnants of embryonic processes that fused in embryogenesis. The midline of the palate is the common location.

The nasopalatine or incisive canal cyst arises from epithelium of the nasopalatine duct. Most common of the fissural cysts, it occurs posterior to and between the roots of the maxillary central incisors. In a periapical film the radiolucency may be heart-shaped (Fig. 5.36). They can become so enlarged as to cause a swelling of the palate. If they arise in the soft tissue, they cause an enlargement of the incisive papilla and are called incisive papilla cysts. The median palatine cyst occurs in the midline of the hard palate. It may or may not appear as a radiolucency mistaken for another cyst until an occlusal radiograph shows the midline radiolucency. As with all of the fissural cysts, the teeth will test vital. The median mandibular cyst is a rare cyst occuring in the midline of the mandible below the apices of the incisors which test vital.

The nonodontogenic cysts of soft tissue are all rare lesions. The nasolabial (nasoalveolar) cyst occurs at the nasolabial fold region as a swelling that obliterates the fold and can appear in the mucolabial fold in-

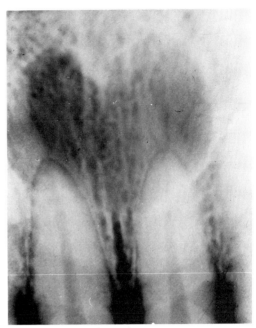

Figure 5.36. Heart-shaped radiolucency characteristic of a nasopalatine cyst.

traorally. Arising probably from nasolacrimal duct epithelium, its location is the soft tissue counterpart of the globulomaxillary cyst.

Lymphoepithelial cysts occur in the lateral neck (branchial cleft cyst) or in the floor of the mouth. They are derived from epithelium proliferating in lymph node tissue, yielding a distinctive pattern and the name. In the neck they may be large and fluctuant swellings mimicking tumors. In the mouth they are small, yellowish lesions resembling pseudocysts and arising in the oral tonsillar tissue (Fig. 5.37). Dermoid cysts occur in the midline and histologically contain keratin and the wall may resemble skin. They may appear above the mylohyoid muscle within the tongue or in the floor of the mouth where they may enlarge and raise up the tongue. Or they may occur below the mylohyoid muscle and appear as a swelling in the submental area. In this area they may resemble the thyroglossal duct cyst, another midline cyst found in the neck (Fig. 5.38) or at the base of the tongue.

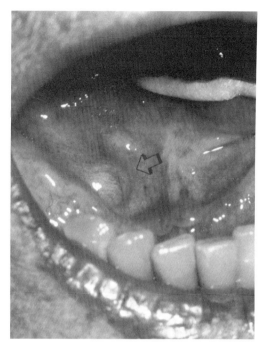

Figure 5.37. Lymphoepithelial cyst, floor of mouth. Clinically, there was a yellow color due to the keratinized cells within the cyst which was arising in an oral tonsil.

Thyroid tissue may be in the wall of these cysts.

The treatment for developmental cysts is local surgical removal or interruption of the cyst wall with ultimate filling in with granulation tissue and restitution of the original tissue.

There are several cyst-like lesions that occur in the jaws, some of which will be mentioned. The traumatic bone "cyst" is an asymptomatic, radiolucent lesion usually of the mandible in the premolar region in a young person (Fig. 5.39). The teeth test vital. When the lesion is surgically explored, an empty sometimes hemorrhagic cavity is found. The lesion heals after the surgery. A history of trauma may or may not be elicited. The lingual mandibular bone concavity (Stafne's bone defect or "cyst") is an anatomical depression on the medial mandibular bone usually posterior and inferior to the mandibular canal appearing as a cystic radiolucency (Fig. 5.40). Not infrequently it occurs anteriorly below the roots of teeth and resembles a cyst. In

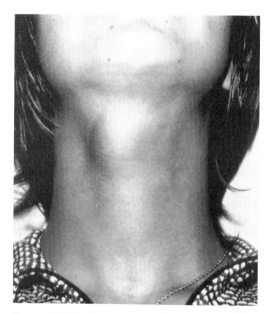

Figure 5.38. Thyroglossal duct cyst. A midline cyst of the neck, there was thyroid tissue in the wall.

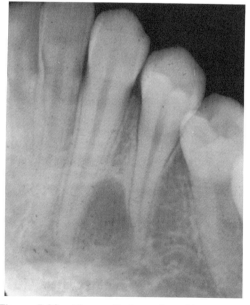

Figure 5.39. Traumatic bone "cyst" in a young person. The teeth were vital. On surgical exploration, there was an empty cavity.

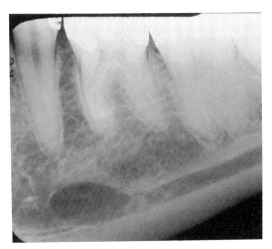

Figure 5.40. Lingual mandibular bone concavity (Stafne's bone defect or "cyst"). The depression, corresponding to the radiolucency, could be palpated on the lingual side of the mandible.

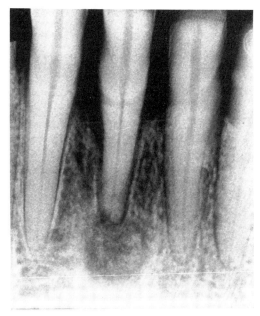

Figure 5.41. Periapical cemental dysplasia, cementoma, at apex of mandibular incisor. Tooth tested vital. Note opacities within radiolucency. No treatment is needed.

the anterior locations the depression may be felt to confirm the diagnosis. A similar condition occurs on the labial side of the maxilla and mandible and is therefore called a labial bone concavity. An example is the cupped out area of the canine fossa in the maxilla. If exaggerated it may resemble a cyst. The osteoporotic marrow defect of bone is a cyst-like radiolucency, usually in the mandible of middle-aged women, in whom there is red marrow replacing mandibular bone. The diagnosis is made after surgical exploration and biopsy of the suspected "cyst".

Periapical cemental dysplasia (cementoma) is a condition in which the bone is replaced by fibrous tissue in which bone or bonelike material can form. Before the bone forms the lesion appears cystic. There is a radiolucency near the apices of usually the mandibular anterior teeth that mimics a periapical inflammatory lesion (Fig. 5.41). However, the teeth test vital and endodontic therapy should be performed. Instead, the lesion(s) are followed radiographically and eventually opacities corresponding to bone are noted within the lesion.

CHAPTER 6

Oral Mucous Membrane Pathology

REVIEW OF NORMAL SKIN AND ORAL MUCOSA

Since the face and oral cavity are constantly under observation by the dental team, some knowledge of the normal histology of the skin and oral mucosa is required to appreciate the changes that can and do occur.

The skin is composed of surface epithelium (epidermis), skin appendages (hair, hair follicles, sweat and sebaceous glands), and the underlying connective tissue (dermis). The epithelium is composed of basically four layers, the stratum basalis or germinal layer, the stratum spinosum or prickle cell layer, the stratum granulosum or granular cell layer, and the corneal or surface layer which is composed of keratin. Beneath the basal layer is a basement membrane area that connects the epithelium to the connective tissue which is composed of collagen fibers.

Normal mucosa is similar to skin in that it also is composed of surface stratified squamous epithelium overlying connective tissue. However, there are several differences between skin and oral mucosa. Whereas skin is always keratinized, the mucosa is mostly parakeratinized. There are essentially three layers of cells in the epithelium (Fig. 6.1). The basal cell layer next to the connective tissue is a single cell layer with the capacity for cell division. Only the basal layer is responsible for the addition of new cells. When cell division does occur, daughter cells cause lateral pressure and "squeeze" other, older, basal cells toward the surface. These cells are then called prickle cells or spinous cells because of the spiny projections seen under the light microscope connecting one cell to the other. This stratum spinosum is several cell layers in thickness. Actually, it is much wider than the spinous cell layer of skin and accounts for the fact that the epithelium of oral mucosa is more than 2 times thicker than the epithelium of skin. In most cases the surface or corneal layer of mucosa contains parakeratin, not keratin. This means that the thin layer of cells at the surface resembles keratin but still retains the nuclei of the cells. Keratin is the tough end product of the squamous epithelial cell. No nuclei are seen in a keratinized layer. In the oral cavity, the attached gingivae, the dorsum of the tongue (papillae) and the hard palate are keratinized. The remaining mucosa is parakeratinized. Keratin tends to give a whiter color to the mucosa because keratin is white clinically. In addition to being mostly parakeratinized and having a thicker epithelium, the mucosa does not have skin appendages. It does, however, contain clusters of accessory salivary glands that secrete mainly mucous on the surface of the mucosa to keep it moist. The major salivary glands—the parotid, the submandibular, and the sublingual—also add to the moist atmosphere of the mucosa. The underlying connective tissue of mucosa is fibrous usually with dense bundles of collagen. There may be some inflammatory cells in the connective tissue, but they are not seen in large numbers. These cells are mainly plasma cells and lymphocytes and indicate that the oral mucosa is constantly warding off foreign agents and bacteria

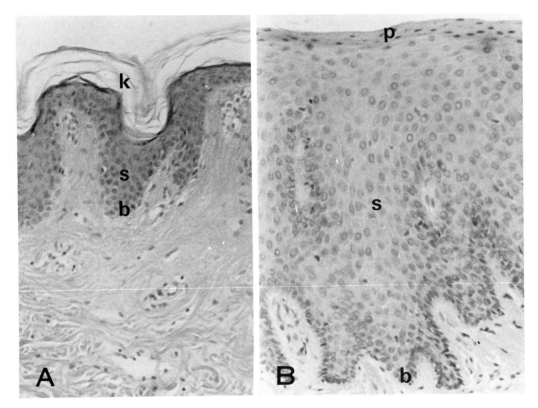

Figure 6.1. *A*, normal skin, and *B*, normal oral mucosa at approximately ×200 magnification. Epithelial cell layers are: *b*, basal; *s*, spinous; *k*, keratin; and *p*, parakeratin.

since these cells are responsible for antigen-antibody type of reactions. The gingival cuff region, in particular, always contains these cells.

The epithelial cells reproduce in the basal cell layers and move toward the surface in a process of maturation by which they become spinous cells and finally keratin or parakeratin. The transit time from the basal cell layer to the time of desquamation is approximately 10–12 days. Thus the mucosa could rebuild itself in about 2 weeks.

The oral mucosa has a great capacity for healing. Coupled with the rapid regeneration time is the fact that it is bathed constantly in saliva. The saliva has antibacterial properties including antibodies, and the moisture it produces results in rapid healing. Therefore, lesions that do not heal in a 2-week period should be suspicious until a proper diagnosis can be made. When the mucosa does heal, it generally does so by regeneration and rarely by scarring. Scars, however, can be seen following deep-seated chronic inflammation, accidents, gingivectomies, and apicoectomies.

BIOPSY

The removal and examination of tissue from the living body is called a biopsy. For many diseases a biopsy is not required for diagnosis. The clinical features may be so characteristic that removal of all or part of the lesion is not necessary. On the other hand, there are times that microscopic examination of tissue will give greater knowledge of a disease and in many instances will allow a definite diagnosis. Biopsy is required whenever a lesion is suspected of being a cancer. A biopsy can confirm or rule out malignancy and is a highly reliable and accurate procedure for this purpose. When additional information is needed to distinguish conditions with similar clinical features, the biopsy is most useful in aiding the diagnosis and approach to treatment. In addition, in cases where the treatment for a known lesion is surgical removal, the surgical specimen should be submitted routinely to confirm the diagnosis. In some cases it may reveal an unsuspected diagnosis.

Biopsy may be either excisional or incisional. Excisional biopsy refers to the surgical removal of the entire lesion plus a surrounding rim of normal tissue. Small lesions are usually removed in this manner (Figs. 6.2–6.4). Incisional biopsy is the removal of only a small portion of the lesion. The site of removal is either sutured or closed or left open to heal. The specimen is placed in a fixative solution, usually 10% neutral buffered formalin, and is submitted along with adequate history and features of the clinical lesion to a diagnostic laboratory. At the laboratory, microscopic slides are prepared for examination by a pathologist.

ORAL CYTOLOGY

Oral exfoliative cytology refers to the scraping of the surface of soft tissue lesions and examination of these cells under a microscope. It is not a substitute for biopsy. It may, however, be useful as an adjunct in diagnosing lesions due to cancer, viruses, fungi, and other diseases. If cytology is used, one must bear in mind that it is not as accurate a test as the biopsy. There is a significant percentage of false negatives occurring in cases relating to cancer detection. If a smear is reported as positive for abnormal cells, a biopsy is mandatory.

The technique for cytology, like the biopsy, is simple and painless. A wooden tongue blade or metal spatula is used to collect the cells from the surface. The tongue blade should be wet with water or saliva. Then the lesion is stroked firmly. The collected cells are smeared on a glass slide with the name of the patient and location of the lesion indicated on the frosted end of the slide. The smeared cells are immediately fixed with hair spray. After drying, the slides and history form are forwarded to a diagnostic laboratory. The slides are stained by the Papanicolaou method and then read as (a) normal cells present—negative for cancer or (b) abnormal cells present (Fig. 6.5). If the latter is true, then a biopsy is mandatory so that adequate treatment is instituted.

MICROSCOPIC CHANGES OF THE ORAL MUCOSA

The microscopic changes seen in the oral mucous membrane consequent to pathologic conditions can be divided into those of the epithelium and those of the connective tissue, for convenience. In reality, there

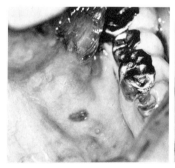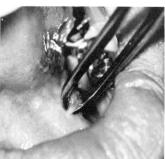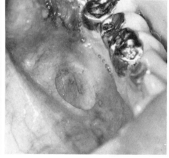

Figure 6.2. *Left*, biopsy of pigmented lesion (amalgam tatoo) from the floor of the mouth.
Figure 6.3. *Middle*, biopsy procedure. Forceps grasp black lesion and some normal tissue. Tissue is cut below forceps.
Figure 6.4. *Right*, biopsy procedure. Black lesion has been removed and placed in formalin fixative. Defect will heal without a suture in this case.

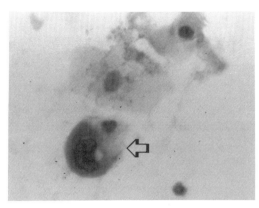

Figure 6.5. Oral cytologic smear of a proven oral cancer. Note positive cancer cell with enlarged nucleus, multiple nucleoli and reversed ratio of nucleus to cytoplasm in contrast to normal squamous cells above.

are changes occurring in both at the same time; however, the change may be more striking in the epithelium or in the connective tissue or even both. The following terms refer to these changes.

Epithelial Changes

Hyperkeratosis refers to an increase or widening in the stratum corneum (Fig. 6.6). This results in excess keratin (hyperorthokeratosis) or parakeratin (hyperparakeratosis) at the surface and yields a white appearance clinically. If the white surface is in the form of a patch, it is called leukoplakia (white patch).

Hyperplasia of the epithelium occurs with the widening or increase in the number of cells in the stratum spinosum (acanthosis). This thickening also would result in a white lesion. Another form of hyperplasia is the extension of rete pegs with their penetration into the connective tissue (Fig. 6.7).

Epithelial dysplasia (dyskeratosis) refers to the abnormal growth pattern or disorientation of the normal layers of epithelium (Fig. 6.8). It generally indicates premalignant changes. The changes can be so severe that they resemble cancer, in which case the term carcinoma in situ is used because

all the cellular characteristics of cancer are present but are confined to the epithelium with no invasion into the connective tissue. This also can be a white or red lesion.

Vesicles can be of two types. Subepithelial vesicles are more common. The accumulation of fluid is beneath the stratum basalis so that all the layers of epithelium are raised (Fig. 6.9). Intraepithelial vesicles are those in which the fluid collects within the epithelial layers, usually the stratum spinosum. The basal layer remains attached to the connective tissue. A rarer type of vesicle, it is important because it can signify the presence of a serious disease, pemphigus. Vesicles rarely are found intact. When they break an ulcer is formed.

An ulcer is a break in the continuity of epithelium. The peripheral epithelium is slightly hyperplastic and clinically shows a rolled margin. The central depressed area without epithelium is covered with a necrotic plug or scab covering granulation tissue. Most often this central portion appears white and the margins are red.

Spongiosis refers to the accumulation of fluid within the cells of the stratum spinosum. This reflects a degeneration of these cells and the microscopic picture resembles a sponge (Fig. 6.10). Clinically, the lesion appears white and is most commonly seen on the buccal mucosa as leukoedema.

Connective Tissue Changes

Inflammatory infiltrates are common. Most often chronic inflammatory cells are present (Fig. 6.11). A prime example is gingivitis.

Hyperplasia of connective tissue refers to an increase in the amount of collagen fibers.

Glandular and ductal distention can be seen in the many accessory mucous glands due to pressure and obstruction.

CLINICAL CHANGES IN THE ORAL MUCOSA

Despite the numerous diseases that can affect the oral mucosa, there are only a

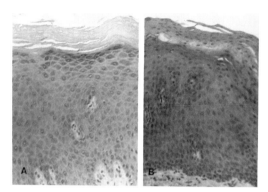

Figure 6.6. *A*, hyperorthokeratosis. Increased thickness of cornified layer with true keratin above granular cell layer. *B*, hyperparakeratosis. Increased thickness of cornified layer with parakeratin (note retained nuclei versus no nuclei in keratin).

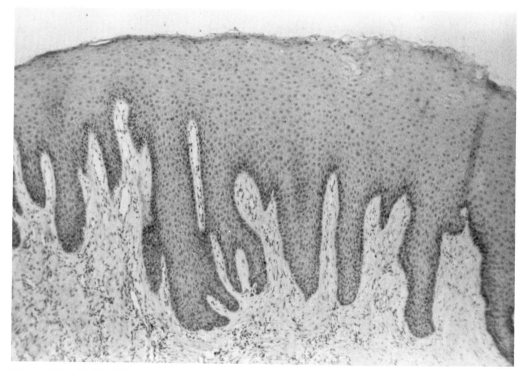

Figure 6.7. Epithelial hyperplasia, an increase in the spinous cell layer, and extension of rete pegs; epithelium extends like fingers into connective tissue.

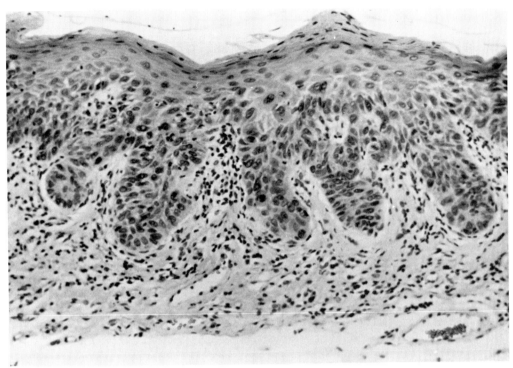

Figure 6.8. Epithelial dysplasia of oral epithelium. Note the haphazard arrangement of cells, particularly in and about the basal cells and drop-shaped rete ridges. The surface shows hyperparakeratosis. This is a premalignant change showing cancer cell changes within the epithelium (magnification ×200).

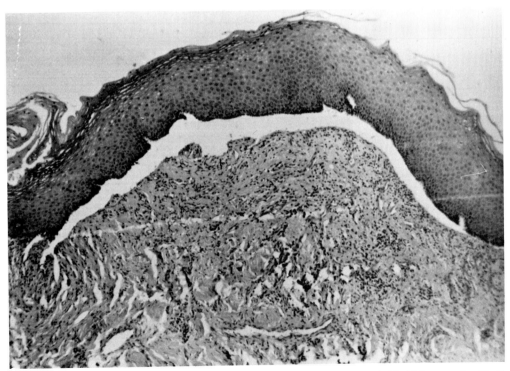

Figure 6.9. Subepithelial vesicle. Space beneath epithelium contained fluid. All layers of epithelium are raised away from connective tissue (magnification ×80).

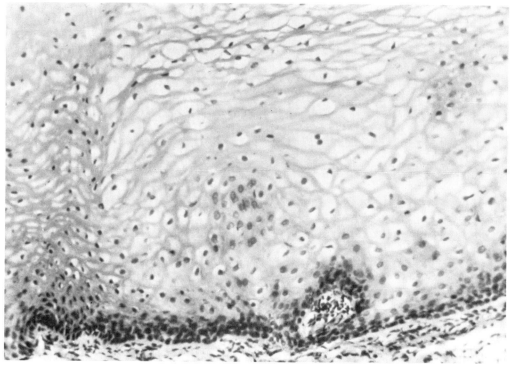

Figure 6.10.   Spongiosis of epithelium. Fluid within epithelial cells gives them the appearance of a sponge (magnification ×200).

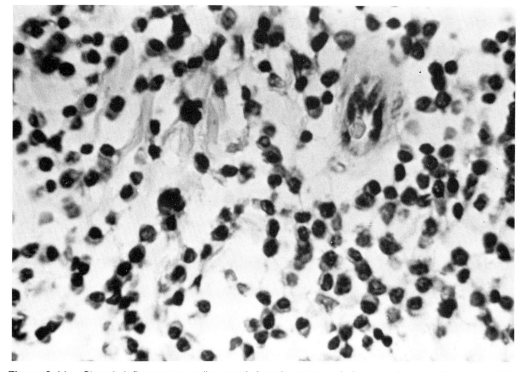

Figure 6.11.   Chronic inflammatory cells, mostly lymphocytes and plasma cells (magnification ×400).

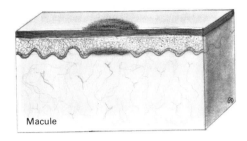

Macule

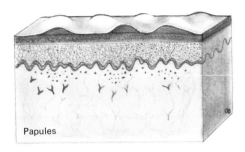

Papules

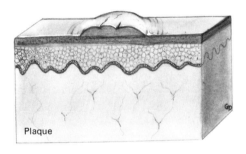

Plaque

limited number of gross lesions that can be seen clinically. A lesion is any wound or pathologic alteration of tissue. Oral mucosal diseases are characterized by one or more lesions that can be categorized into these basic types: macule, papule, plaque, vesicle, bulla, ulcer, erosion, nodule, tumor, atrophic area, scar, and crust (Figs. 6.12, 6.18, 6.23). The recognition of these lesions is of prime importance for unless these are noted, oral disease will be overlooked.

A *macule* or macula is a flat spot, stain, or blemish on the mucosa (Fig. 6.13). It varies in size and color and may be red, blue, black, or another color. Examples are the common amalgam tatoo (Fig. 6.2), melanin pigmentation of a nevus, the rash of secondary syphilis, or a small area of hemorrhage, a petechia.

A *papule* or papula is a small, rounded, pimple-like, variably colored elevation. They usually appear in clumps and are commonly seen in lichen planus in which they appear as white elevations with variable patterns (Fig. 6.14).

A *plaque* is a small or large, demarcated patch that can be smooth or fissured (Fig. 6.15). Leukoplakia refers to a white patch or plaque. The leukoplakia may represent simple hyperkeratosis, dysplasia, or cancer. Erythroplasia is a red patch. It tends to be flat rather than raised and is usually malignant or premalignant unless it is associated with another known disease. It must be differentiated from a rash.

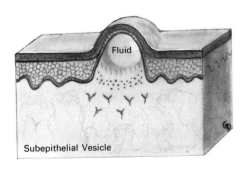

Subepithelial Vesicle

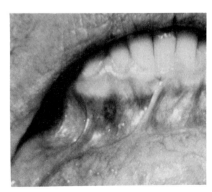

Figure 6.12. Diagrams of oral mucosal changes.

Figure 6.13. Black macule, unattached gingiva. Carbon tattoo from a pencil.

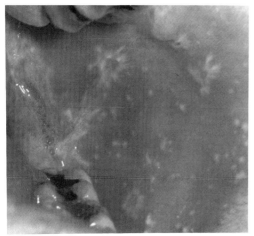

Figure 6.14. Lichen planus. There are white, keratotic, nonremovable papules, some of which form patterns.

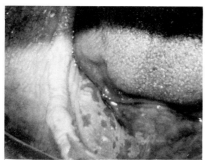

Figure 6.15. Leukoplakia (white patch), buccal mucosa, alveolar ridge, and floor of mouth.

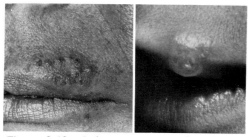

Figure 6.16. *Left*, numerous small vesicles on the skin of the upper lip (herpes labialis).
Figure 6.17. *Right*, several vesicles have coalesced to form a large vesicle or bulla on the upper lip (herpes labialis).

A *vesicle* is a small bleb or blister representing accumulation of fluid beneath or within the epithelium (Fig. 6.16). Clinically, the subepithelial type cannot be dis-

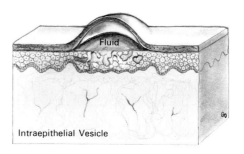

Intraepithelial Vesicle

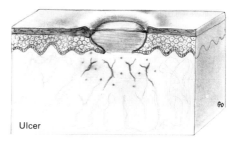

Ulcer

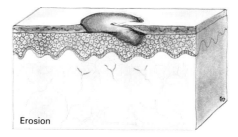

Erosion

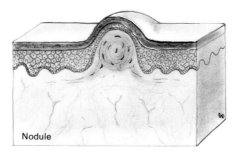

Nodule

Figure 6.18. Diagrams of oral mucosal changes.

tinguished from the intraepithelial. Viral diseases cause vesicles to form. Intact vesicles are commonly seen in herpes labialis of the lips. However, within the oral cavity intact vesicles are rarely seen because they are traumatized readily. Once a vesicle is traumatized or the membrane is ruptured spontaneously, an ulcer is formed.

A *bulla* is merely a large vesicle or blister (Fig. 6.17). It may form when several vesicles coalesce. Pemphigus and drug reactions are characterized by bullae. The bulla may appear white due to the necrosis of the overlying degenerating epithelium (Fig. 6.19).

An *ulcer* is a sore characterized by the loss of epithelium yielding a punched out shallow or deep area. The central zone of necrosis appears as a white or yellowish membrane and is surrounded by a red halo (Fig. 6.20). They may be large or small and

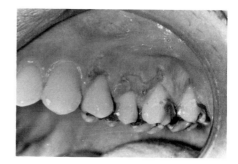

Figure 6.21. Erosion and ulcer of traumatic origin (toothbrush). Erosion is red area on gingiva over the first bicuspid.

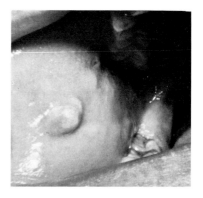

Figure 6.22. Nodule on buccal mucosa (fibroma).

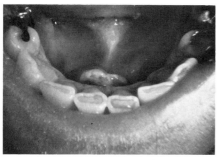

Figure 6.19. Bulla, floor of the mouth. Surface is degenerative and appears white (pemphigus).

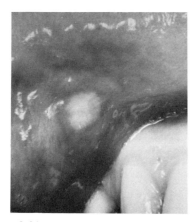

Figure 6.20. Ulcer, inner aspect upper lip (aphthous stomatitis).

the border may be hard and raised. Traumatic ulcers are the most common. Ulcers are also seen in aphthous stomatitis, cancer, and tuberculosis.

An *erosion* of the mucosa refers to the partial loss of the upper layers of the epithelium. These lesions appear red because the blood supply in the connective tissue can be seen easier in the area where there is less epithelium. Examples of mucosal erosions are traumatic erosion caused by toothbrushing (Fig. 6.21) and a form of lichen planus called erosive lichen planus. These lesions appear as red, raw denuded areas.

A *nodule* is a localized swelling or protuberance. It is usually solid, raised and firm and can measure from millimeters to centimeters. It usually represents a growth from the connective tissue. A common example is the fibroma (Fig. 6.22). Mucosal cysts and cystlike masses are specialized nodules in that they are not firm. A mucocele of the lip presents as a nodular mass.

A *tumor* is a swelling of a part. It could be inflammatory but often is considered as a developmental or neoplastic solid growth projecting outward and arising from the mucosa. A hemangioma is a benign tumor (Fig. 6.24). Carcinoma or cancer is a malignant tumor (Fig. 6.25).

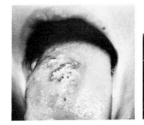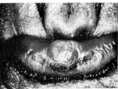

Figure 6.24. *Left*, benign tumor involving over half the tongue (hemangioma).
Figure 6.25. *Right*, malignant tumor of the lower lip (carcinoma).

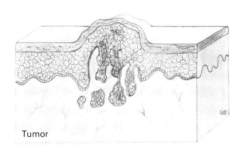

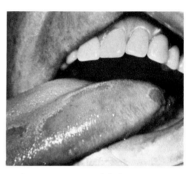

Figure 6.26. Atrophy of filiform papillae due to denture trauma caused large red denuded area on left lateral border of tongue. A lesion of geographic tongue appears at posterior lateral border.

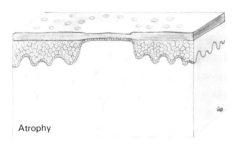

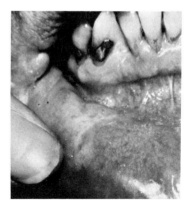

Figure 6.27. Scars, inner aspect lower lip (healed, deep aphthous ulcers).

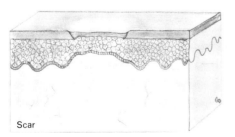

Figure 6.23. Diagrams of oral mucosal changes.

Atrophy refers to reddened areas of the mucosa where the epithelium is thin and the blood supply of the connective tissue is seen (Fig. 6.26). It differs from erosion in that there are less cells in the epithelium due to atrophy of the epithelium, not because of trauma. Examples of atrophy would be seen in geographic tongue where the filiform papillae are lost as well as in vitamin deficiency states, anemias, and tertiary syphilis.

A *scar* is a white depressed mark, line, or area that represents healing after injury. It is rare in the oral cavity, but is seen following gingivectomies, apicoectomies, and deep inflammation. Scars are frequently seen on the lips (Fig. 6.27), mucosa, and skin surface as reminders of previous trauma.

A *crust* is a scab or dry outer layer. It is usually seen with brown pigmentation of the skin or outer surface of the lips (Fig. 6.28). A scab in the mouth is white and is represented by the central white necrotic area of an ulcer.

VIRAL INFECTIONS OF THE ORAL CAVITY

Viruses are the smallest of microorganisms that can produce infection. Infection is the invasion of tissue by pathologic microorganisms with resulting damage to the tissue, inflammation, and systemic involvement. Viruses are smaller than bacteria, can be isolated by special technique, and observed by electron microscopy. They are composed of an outer protein coating surrounding an inner core of either ribonucleic acid (RNA) or deoxyribonucleic acid (DNA). Found everywhere, they infect animals, plants, and bacteria. They live within cells and utilize the cell's metabolic machinery for their own reproduction. Characteristically, they choose specific cells of the body. This tendency to turn to, to choose, or to have an affinity for certain cells and not others is called tropism. Viruses, then, can be categorized according to the tissue that is mainly involved or infected.

Dermotropic viruses select the skin and mucous membranes. Included in this group are the viruses that cause chickenpox, smallpox, measles, and the herpes simplex virus, which involves mainly the mouth.

Pneumotropic viruses affect the respiratory system and are responsible for the common cold and influenza.

Neurotropic viruses involve nerve tissue. Herpes zoster, encephalitis, rabies, and poliomyelitis are diseases caused by these viruses.

Glandulotropic viruses infect glands. Mumps of the parotid gland is an example.

Oral involvement by viruses is very common. The disease may affect only the mouth or the oral mucosa may be involved concurrent with spread of infection from other parts that are infected. Those infections confined to the mouth are herpetic stomatitis (stomato—mouth), herpes labialis, and herpangina. Those that include both the skin and the mouth are chickenpox, measles, mumps, and herpes zoster.

Usually, once an individual is infected with a virus, the defense system of the body reacts. Lymphocytes recognize the virus as foreign and plasma cells produce neutralizing antibodies against it to overcome the infection. Characteristically, for most viruses, the immunity to further infection is long lasting. However, important exceptions to this are the common cold virus and the herpes simplex virus and the chickenpox virus.

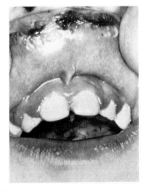

Figure 6.28. Crusts on upper lip (herpetic stomatitis).

Primary Herpetic Stomatitis
(Acute Herpetic Gingivostomatitis)

Herpetic stomatitis may follow the primary contact with the herpes simplex virus. Maternal antibodies offer protection for about 6 months. After this the child (age 3–10 usually), young adult, or even adult becomes infected on exposure. Following exposure there is an incubation period common to all viral diseases. This represents the interval between the moment of exposure and the manifestation of the disease. With a first exposure to herpes simplex, two courses are possible. In most individuals, the disease is subclinical, meaning that antibodies are produced but no signs and symptoms of the disease appear. In about 10% of the population, individuals manifest the disease. Although the virus can affect the skin, the vagina, the conjunctiva, and the meninges, it most commonly manifests as a disease state of the oral cavity.

After the incubation period in the patient, there is a prodromal period in which there are symptoms signifying the onset of the disease. The patient suddenly feels ill and runs a high fever. Swelling and pain appear in the mouth. Then, characteristically, vesicles develop. These may occur anywhere in the oral cavity. They may be few or scattered. Some may coalesce and form a bulla. The vesicles soon rupture and form ulcers with a red halo (Figs. 6.29 and 6.30). The vesicles form because the replication of the herpes virus within the cells causes degeneration and death of epithelial cells. This initiates an inflammatory reaction and fluid collects to form the vesicle. The vesicles may continue to develop for a week, but within 10–14 days all lesions disappear, and the mucosa heals without scarring and appears normal.

Besides the vesicular eruptions, there are other manifestations. The gingivae are intensely inflamed and appear red both on the marginal and attached gingivae (Fig. 6.31). In addition, the tongue, besides having eruptions, is usually coated and appears white, a feature common in viral infections and fevers (Fig. 6.32). The fungiform papillae may be prominent due to the edema. The lips also are swollen, and have vesicles that soon rupture leaving ulcers which appear as crusts. Lymph nodes are usually swollen and tender.

The disease runs a course of about 2 weeks. The build-up of antibodies is coexistent with the disappearance of the symptoms and lesions. The treatment is therefore to treat the symptoms. The mouth is generally so sore that patients cannot eat. A soothing mouthwash, aspirin for fever, and bed rest are prescribed. Antibiotics are

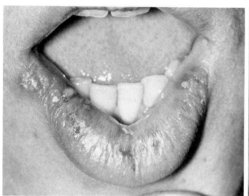 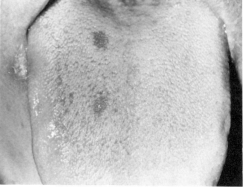

Figure 6.29. *Left*, herpetic stomatitis, 24-year-old female. Many vesicles have ruptured leaving discrete ulcers with halos on lower lip.

Figure 6.30. *Right*, herpetic stomatitis, same patient as in Figure 6.29. Note intact small vesicle below, and atrophic area of ruptured vesicle, above. Tongue is uniformly coated and whitened.

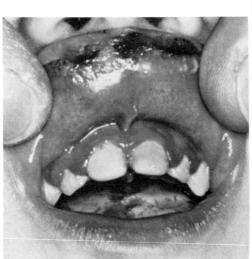 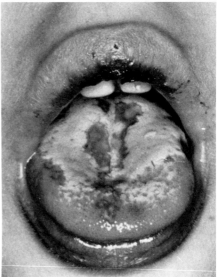

Figure 6.31. *Left,* primary herpetic gingivostomatitis, 9-year-old male. Gingivae uniformly reddened. Lips are crusted.
Figure 6.32. *Right,* primary herpetic gingivostomatitis, same as Figure 6.31. Note many ulcers on white-coated tongue.

ineffective against viruses and are not used for viral infections unless there is evidence of secondary bacterial infection.

Usually the antibody response confers immunity against another attack of the primary disease. However, despite the antibodies, some individuals may have a secondary disease. One affects the intraoral tissues, the other the lips. After the primary infection, the virus remains dormant. In the head area it is in the trigeminal ganglion. By an unknown triggering mechanism, the virus is reactivated and spreads along the nerve pathway to produce vesicles in epithelium at a peripheral location. Factors associated with the outbreak of lesions are trauma, emotions, fever, infections, menstruation, and allergy—among others.

Recurrent Intraoral Herpes Simplex

These are called recurrent herpetic ulcers because the vesicles are rarely seen intact. The manifestations of these recurrent episodes are in no way as dramatic as the primary disease. Usually, there is a prodromal symptom of tingling or slight pain, followed by the eruption of a vesicle which soon ruptures. The resulting ulcers are small but may be large if several vesicles coalesce. Characteristically, they occur on bound down or firmly attached mucosa, such as the hard palate and attached gingivae, and not movable mucosa (Fig. 6.33). (This is important in distinguishing the herpetic ulcer from an aphthous ulcer.) A cytologic smear in the early phases often shows swollen, distorted nuclei of affected epithelial cells. The ulcers heal in about 7 days. No treatment is required unless symptoms demand it.

Herpes Labialis
(Recurrent Herpes Labialis)

Herpes labialis (cold sores) is the more common of the recurrent herpetic infections. Some of the precipitating factors are the common cold, febrile diseases, and exposure to direct sunlight, which have lead to the names of common usage of cold sores, fever blisters, and sun blisters, respectively.

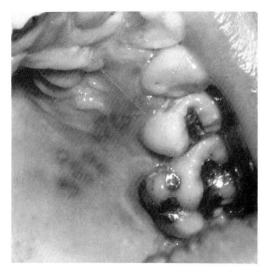

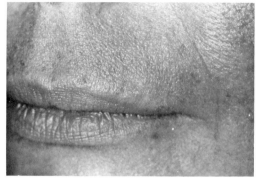

Figure 6.34–6.38. Sequence photographs.
Figure 6.34. Herpes labialis, upper lip, day 1: prodromal stage, tingling, following exposure to sun.

Figure 6.33. Recurrent intraoral herpes of hard palate. Note small, punctate, clustered ulcers. The patient felt a burning before the outbreak of vesicles.

The disease starts with prodromal symptoms such as a tingling or burning sensation in the lip at the future site of the vesicles (Figs. 6.34–6.38). Within 24 hours small vesicles appear in clusters usually on the skin surface of the lips, upper or lower. There may be á few or many vesicles (Fig. 6.39). Some may coalesce to form a bulla (Fig. 6.40). The vesicles rupture leaving ulcers which crust on the skin surface and appear brown. There may be extensive edema, with redness and swelling (Fig. 6.41). The ulcers heal usually in 5–7 days and leave no scars. Scratching can spread the infection. The disease runs its course and can heal without treatment. However, herpes labialis is extremely annoying and tends to recur in the same individuals repeatedly. Dabbing the site with 70% isopropyl alcohol prior to blistering may dry out the vesicles. Treatment is variable. Most clinicians attempt to shorten the course of the disease. Some antiviral drugs are available but have restricted usage. Vaccines will be available and offer the greatest hope for prevention and cure. For the dental team there should be precautions taken so that

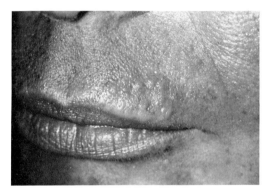

Figure 6.35. Herpes labialis, day 2: vesicles at site of tingling.

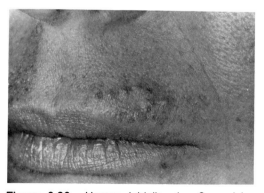

Figure 6.36. Herpes labialis, day 3: vesicles have begun to weep and ulcerate.

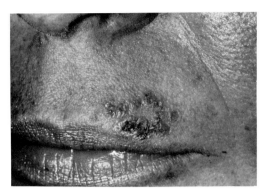

Figure 6.37.   Herpes labialis, day 5: ulcers have crusted.

the herpetic infection is not transmitted to the fingers (herpetic whitlow).

Herpangina

Herpangina is a viral disease caused by strains of the Coxsackie virus. In particular it affects the posterior part of the mouth. There is a prodromal period of fever and ill

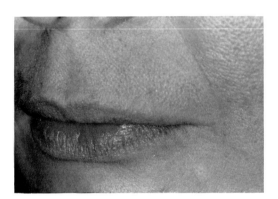

Figure 6.38.   Herpes labialis, day 7: skin healed, normal.

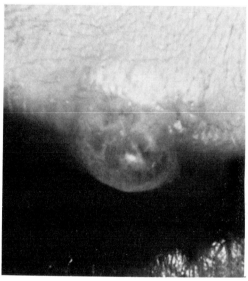

Figure 6.40.   Herpes labialis, upper lip. Several vesicles have coalesced to form a large blister.

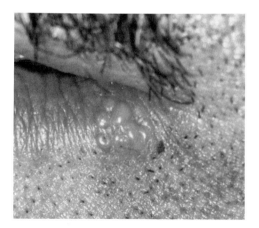

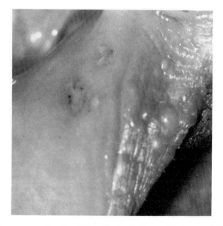

Figure 6.39.   Recurrent herpes labialis due to the trauma of a lip bite. Note *left*, multiple vesicles on skin side of lower lip; and *right*, corresponding ulcer on inner lip.

feeling. Following this, groups of vesicles appear mainly on the soft palate and tonsillar areas. The vesicles will then rupture. Patients complain of a severe sore throat which may be confused with a "strep throat." The disease runs its course in 7–10 days. Only symptomatic treatment is required.

Herpes Zoster

Herpes zoster (shingles) is a viral disease caused by a reactivation of the chickenpox

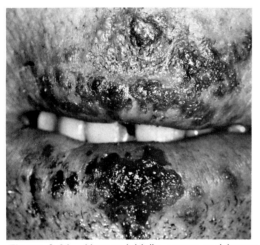

Figure 6.41. Herpes labialis, upper and lower lips, after only one exposure to sun. There are several vesicles, ulcers, crusts, and extensive swelling and edema.

(varicella) virus. Occurring in older or immunosuppressed individuals the disease erupts along peripheral nerves leading from the dorsal root ganglion where the virus was dormant. Starting as pain the disease manifests itself by painful vesicular eruptions on the skin but may affect the oral cavity when the trigeminal (Vth cranial nerve) is infected. The vesicular eruption in herpes zoster is striking because it is unilateral. For instance, when it affects the trigeminal nerve, the eruptions appear on the skin only on one side of the face and on one side of the mouth (palate, tongue) outlining the distribution of the nerves (Figs. 6.42 and 6.43). The disease runs a course of weeks and months without treatment and pain may linger after lesions heal.

Other viruses affecting the skin also may have vesicular eruptions in the mouth but the oral eruptions are secondary features. Chickenpox (varicella) and measles (rubeola) are exanthematous viral diseases of childhood usually characterized by vesicles and fever. Some vesicles may appear in the mouth. The Koplik spots of measles are supposed to appear on the buccal mucosa 24 hours before the outbreak of the disease. Clinicians, however, are hard pressed to find and prove the existence of these spots.

Occasionally, on examination, one may find a single vesicle on the soft palate.

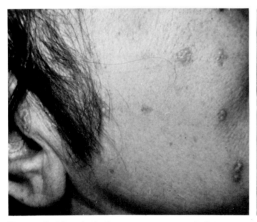 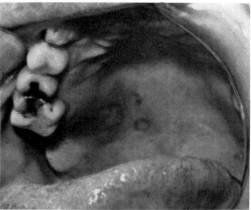

Figure 6.42. *Left*, herpes zoster, painful vesicular eruptions on right side of face along mandibular branch of trigeminal nerve.
Figure 6.43. *Right*, herpes zoster, same patient as in Figure 6.42. Note unilateral distribution of ulcers on right palate. Ulcers started as vesicles.

Follow-up of these cases shows that the patient has a cold or is about to get one. The vesicle represents an attack by a pneumotropic virus.

Mumps is a glandular viral disease usually affecting the parotid gland. High fever is followed by a painful swelling behind the ear. The papilla to the parotid (Stensen's) duct may be swollen and the secretions of the parotid are lessened so the mouth may be dry. The pain subsides but the swelling persists for about 5 days and then abates. The submandibular and sublingual glands may also be affected. The facial swelling can mimic a cellulitis (Fig. 6.44).

Infectious mononucleosis, caused by the *Herpesvirus*, Epstein-Barr virus, manifests with swollen neck nodes, a sore throat and abnormal blood monocytes. The palatine tonsils are frequently involved and in the early stages may resemble "strep throat" (Fig. 6.45). The tonsils become greatly enlarged and necrotic. Petechiae of the palate may be noted. There is no effective treatment. The disease may last for months and involve the liver.

It is to be noted that viral diseases manifest themselves mainly with the eruption of vesicles when they involve the oral cavity. However, other conditions may cause vesicular eruptions. Among these are drug reactions, allergies and several dermatologic-oral diseases. In addition, because the vesicles rupture and leave ulcers, it may be difficult at times to label them as viral ulcers. Other ulcerative conditions must then be considered.

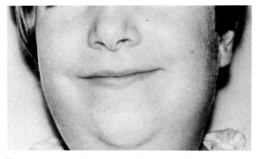

Figure 6.44. Facial swelling in a 7-year-old female who had mumps for 4 days when this photo was taken.

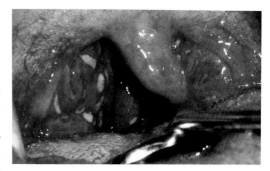

Figure 6.45. Infectious mononucleosis, early phase. Positive serologic tests. Swollen palatine tonsils with necrotic material in crypts in an 18-year-old with sore throat and posterior neck adenopathy. A "strep throat" would look similar.

Aphthous Stomatitis (Recurrent Aphthous Stomatitis: Canker Sores)

Aphtha means small ulcer or white spot. The common disease of aphthous stomatitis is characterized by one or more usually small, painful ulcers affecting the movable or mucous gland-bearing mucosa. The small ulcers often resemble those formed by the rupture of a herpetic vesicle, showing as a white spot with a red halo. Thus the two diseases may be confused. However, aphthous stomatitis is not a viral disease. The aphthae do not arise from vesicles. There are etiologic as well as precipitating factors.

A streptococcal organism *Streptococcus sanguis*, of the normal oral flora, has been isolated as an agent causing this disease. There appears to be a localized immune response against this organism as well as to the epithelium of the host. The ensuing inflammatory response causes localized damage to the host in the form of degeneration and necrosis. The overlying epithelium loses its blood supply and an ulcer is formed. Invariably in patients with aphthous stomatitis, there is a recall of some emotionally stressful event associated antecedent to the formation of the ulcer. For this reason, aphthous stomatitis is considered one of the psychosomatic diseases. Other precipitating factors are trauma, hormonal changes as menses, and allergy to foods. Some nutritional deficiencies manifest with canker-like ulcers.

Patients give a history of some sensation such as tingling at the site of the future ulcer. Then a red macule appears. This is followed by the breakdown of the epithelium (ulceration). The ulcers are characteristic with a central white or yellow area surrounded by a halo of erythema (Fig. 6.46). They appear punched out, usually oval or round, but may be linear. The ulcers may be singular or multiple (Fig. 6.47). They can occur anywhere in the mouth and lips. In contrast to recurrent intraoral herpetic ulcers, aphthous ulcers occur on the unattached and movable mucosa. Small ulcers are called minor aphthae. Large, longstanding ones are major aphthae and heal by scarring. Some ulcers may coexist with genital ulcers (Behçet's syndrome). Some patients may have only one episode whereas others may have recurrent attacks. The intervals vary from years to months. Some individuals are never free of the ulcers, with a new one appearing as the older one(s) heals. Thus a history of recurrence is significant for diagnosis. All age groups can be affected but the incidence is highest in young adults. The ulcers are extremely painful so that the patient often seeks aid.

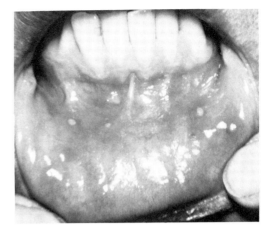

Figure 6.47. Aphthous stomatitis. Multiple discrete small ulcers on labial mucosa. They resemble herpetic ulcers; however, note gingivae are not involved.

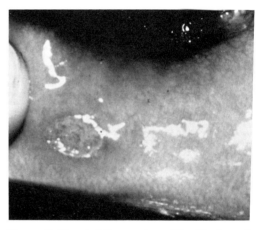

Figure 6.48. Aphthous stomatitis. Healing ulcer. Necrotic area is being replaced by new epithelial surface.

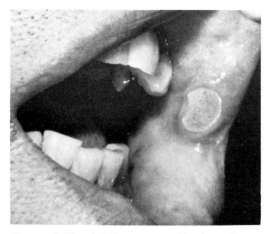

Figure 6.46. Aphthous stomatitis, buccal mucosa near commissure. A large ulcer with oval white central area surrounded by a wide zone of erythema. This was extremely painful.

Treatment varies with the severity of the lesions and the attitude of the patients. Tetracycline mouth rinses, topical corticosteroids and anesthetic mouth rinses are effective. Wiping off the scab and using hydrogen peroxide work well. Sometimes, systemic steroids are used. However, there are no curative measures to date. The small ulcers will heal unaided in 5–14 days. A very large ulcer will take months. Minor aphthae usually heal without scarring, but major aphthae with deep inflammation heal with a scar (Figs. 6.48 and 6.49).

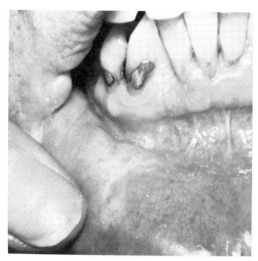

Figure 6.49. Aphthous stomatitis. Deep, long-standing ulcers have healed by scarring of the labial mucosa.

The clinical appearance of ulcers in aphthous stomatitis is sufficiently characteristic that the term aphthous ulcer is often used. An ulcer with the typical aphthous characteristics coupled with a history of pain and recurrence probably represents aphthous stomatitis. However, there are many other conditions with ulcerations which must be considered possibilities before a final diagnosis is made.

Besides ulcerations of viral, drug, or allergic background, there are the common ulcers produced by trauma. These traumatic ulcers become infected secondarily by oral bacteria and therefore can be considered bacterial infections. Traumatic ulcers and traumatic lesions of the oral mucosa are extremely common, and trauma should be considered first when ulcers, erosions, and atrophic areas are noted.

The trauma may be mechanical, chemical, thermal, or electrical, the most common being mechanical. This includes lacerations and abrasions by many objects, such as teeth, restorations, dental procedures, and foreign objects. A badly decayed tooth often has sharp edges of enamel that tear the mucosa (Fig. 6.50). Dental prostheses and worn restorations may have sharp edges. Orthodontic appliances frequently cause ulcerations. Accidental biting of the mucosa causes painful sores. Any sharp object introduced into the mouth by the patient, hygienist, or dentist can create trauma. Trauma may be induced by the patient (factitial trauma), in which case a careful inquiry will elicit that history. Ill-fitting dentures are a common source of traumatic lesions, one of which is the traumatic ulcer.

Traumatic ulcers vary according to the nature of the cause, the duration of the infliction, and the amount of secondary bacterial invasion. Generally, they are discreet ulcers, with a punched-out appearance. The shape can vary and often the borders are jagged. Like other ulcers, the central necrotic zone is white and there is a variable red halo surrounding it. They can be painful, but pain is not always a prominent feature as it is with aphthous ulcers. They heal within 7–10 days usually depending on the size and the removal of the source of the problem. The cause is usually quite apparent either through history or through examination. For example, toothbrush abrasion with erosions and ulcerations is frequently seen because patients are overzealous about brushing prior to appointments (Fig. 6.51). A newly placed denture often results in ulcerations. When the denture is relined the ulcers heal un-

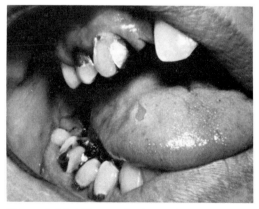

Figure 6.50. Traumatic ulcer on tongue. Patient rubbed tongue over sharp edges of buccal surface of decayed molar.

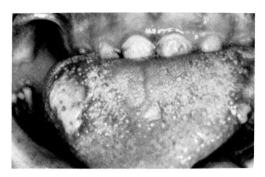

Figure 6.51. Traumatic ulcers of tongue and buccal mucosa, caused by overzealous toothbrushing in a youngster. Ulcers have a thick white necrotic pseudomembrane.

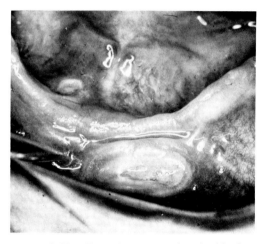

Figure 6.52. Two ulcers associated with denture trauma. When denture was withheld from patient, the large ulcer on the labial sulcus healed, but the smaller ulcer on the lingual sulcus did not. Biopsy proved it to be a squamous cell carcinoma.

eventfully. Conversely, an ill-fitting denture moves and cuts into the mucosa. Relining or remaking the denture is required to alleviate the problem. Thus, therapy for the traumatic ulcer depends on the symptoms and on finding and removing the cause. If an ulcer fails to heal within 2 weeks, then it should be suspected of being cancer until proven otherwise (Fig. 6.52).

There are other traumatic lesions produced by dentures. A traumatic glossitis-appearing geographic tongue may be seen on the lateral border of the tongue. The lingual surface is devoid of filiform papillae and atrophic and appears red, swollen, and shiny. The cause is the abrasion of the tongue against the lingual surfaces of the denture teeth either by neurotic habit or poor alignment of the teeth. The atrophic areas do not change as they do with geographic tongue.

Denture sore mouth is another condition related to dentures. The palate, maxillary, and mandibular ridges in particular appear bright red, swollen, and often are burning and painful. The cause appears to be poorly adapted dentures. It is treated with soft tissue-relining material until healing occurs, then new dentures are constructed. Sometimes a fungal infection, candidiasis, is associated with denture sore mouth.

Chemical trauma is caused by the application of drugs or burning chemical to the mucosa. An aspirin burn can be caused by placing aspirins against a painful tooth, a practice that should be discouraged. The aspirin, being acid, burns the mucosa and leaves a white pseudomembrane representing the necrotic epithelium (Fig. 6.53). The white membrane can be removed leaving a raw ulcer. Other chemicals include household items such as lye that can cause severe burns. Mouthwashes, if used in full strength over a sufficient period of time, can cause chemical erosion and burns. Some toothpastes due to the preservatives

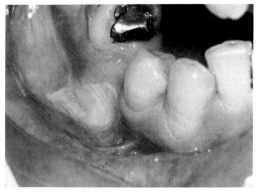

Figure 6.53. Aspirin burn, right buccal vestibule. The acid has coagulated the epithelium causing a white lesion.

also have this capability. Silver nitrate, a cauterizing and disinfecting agent, will burn and necrotize mucosa when it is applied.

Thermal injury can also cause severe damage to the mucosa. The most common examples are those caused by hot food or liquids taken into the mouth (Fig. 6.54). Soups frequently cause burns on the lips and the mucosa appears white and may form a vesicle. Hot cheese, as in grilled sandwiches and pizza is a common offender. The pizza burn usually occurs on the palate. The lesion is a striking, irregular, white-yellow slough with underlying ulceration. The pain may be severe. Ointments may help alleviate the discomfort and aid healing which takes about 10 days to 2 weeks.

Electrical burns are rare with exception of those purposefully done as part of therapy utilizing electrosurgery or electrocautery. A child biting into an electrical cord may get a severe irregular burn, with white slough on the lip. Treatment in this case would include plastic surgery.

There are other common lesions of the mucosa related to irritation and trauma that can also be considered as nonspecific bacterial infections. The oral flora is that group of bacteria that are normally present in the mouth and usually are nonpathogenic. These flora may exaggerate traumatic lesions, ulcers, and other conditions. The lesions listed below are at one time or another involved with these bacteria. Because there are many bacteria and no single microbial agent responsible, these infections are called nonspecific. In addition, because of their clinical appearance these same lesions can be considered tumor-like because they are essentially swellings and resemble some tumors. In fact, however, they are inflammatory responses to irritation. The inflammation is long-standing, though, and so the component of hyperplasia is present and responsible for the tumor-like appearance.

Most of the time these inflammatory hyperplastic overgrowths occur on the gingivae. Therefore, they have been called epulides. An epulis is a swelling of the gingiva. Although most are caused by local irritation and may look alike, they have different names, depending on the microscopic diagnosis. Thus, an epulis may be: a pyogenic granuloma, a peripheral fibroma, a peripheral ossifying fibroma, a peripheral giant cell granuloma, a hemangioma, or granulation tissue, depending on the microscopic pattern.

The pyogenic granuloma is a common lesion that usually occurs on the labial gingiva, although it can occur anywhere in the mouth. Clinically, it is a nodular, raised, rounded mass with a red to purple hue often with scattered white masses representing ulcerative zones. Bacteria are involved with these surface ulcerations and originally were thought to be the causative agent. (Pyogenic refers to pus-producing organisms.) The growth is, in fact, an overgrowth of granulation tissue, accounting for the red color and for the ease of bleeding. The treatment is surgical removal; sometimes the lesions recur (Fig. 6.55).

Pregnancy tumors are pyogenic granulomas that occur on the gingiva of pregnant women. They have the same clinical appearance and undoubtedly are responses to local irritation. The gingiva in pregnant women can have an exaggerated response

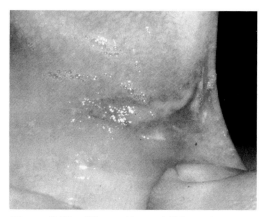

Figure 6.54. Thermal burn, left buccal mucosa, caused by hot fork. Necrotic epithelium and scab appear white.

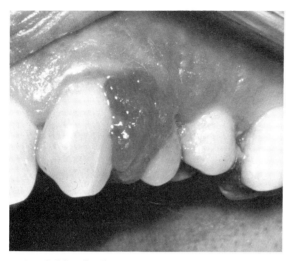
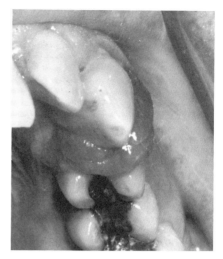

Figure 6.55. Epulis. Microscopically, a pyogenic granuloma. This red lesion grew rapidly and bled easily (two views of same patient).

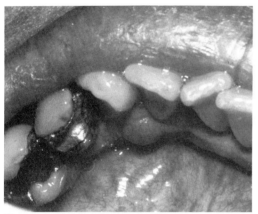
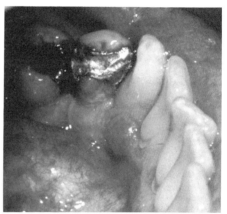

Figure 6.56. Epulis, gingiva lingual to mandibular canine and lateral incisor. A peripheral giant cell granuloma, this was blue-purple like a hemangioma (two views of same patient).

to irritants such as calculus. Unless the lesions are particularly bothersome, they are effectively removed following delivery. They are not true tumors and are not premalignant.

Following the extraction of teeth, there may be an exuberant inflammatory response in the socket site. Not infrequently a lesion similar to the pyogenic granuloma is seen protruding from the socket like a raspberry. These are called epulis granulomatosa or granulation tissue and often foreign bodies are noted within them. They bleed readily. Simple surgical removal is the treatment.

Peripheral giant cell granuloma or giant cell epulis is a red, blue, raised, firm swelling occurring only on the gingiva (Fig. 6.56). It resembles the pyogenic granuloma and differs only histologically in that numerous giant cells are found scattered throughout the granulation tissue. It appears suddenly and rapidly increases in size. Treatment is surgical removal. They also may recur. The term peripheral is used because there is a similar histologic lesion that can occur within the jaw, in which instance it is termed central giant cell granuloma. When in the bone there is a cystic appearance on the radiograph.

Besides the denture ulcer, an ill-fitting denture is responsible for two common hyperplastic and tumor-like lesions. Epulis fissuratum or denture hyperplasia repre-

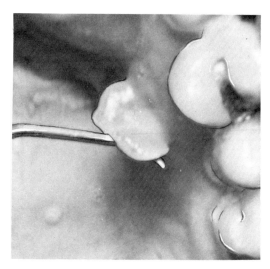

Figure 6.59. Denture hyperplasia. Inflammatory growth associated with a temporary acrylic appliance used to replace missing anterior incisors.

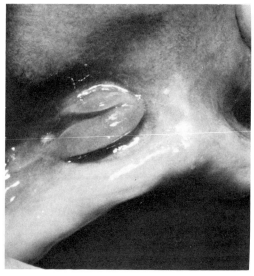

Figure 6.57. Epulis fissuratum, denture hyperplasia. Growth of tissue in labial sulcus corresponding to position of denture flange that caused the trauma.

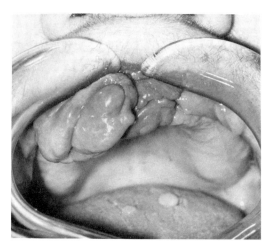

Figure 6.58. Epulis fissuratum, extensive overgrowth of flabby tissue related to poorly fitting denture.

sents the reaction of the tissue at the flanges or peripheral borders of a loose denture (FIgs. 6.57–6.59). The tissue appears as red, flabby, grooved folds, running along the margins of the denture. Often the patients give a history of not having had an adjustment of the denture when it was first inserted. It is also often seen when the patient has a maxillary denture and mandibular anterior teeth but no posterior teeth. Then every time the patient bites, the mandibular anterior teeth cause the maxillary denture to move in the anterior area thus producing the hyperplastic tissue. With an overextended margin, an ulcer develops. If the denture is not corrected, the long-standing inflammation and continued trauma lead to the excess of tissue. The overgrowth is of both the epithelium and connective tissue which is usually quite vascular, accounting for the red color. The treatment is surgical removal of the redundant folds and fabrication of a new properly fitting denture.

Inflammatory papillary hyperplasia or papillary hyperplasia of the palate refers to a reddened palate with numerous small pebble-like projections or nodules much like a raspberry (Fig. 6.60). It occurs mainly

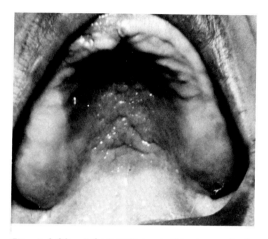

Figure 6.60. Inflammatory papillary hyperplasia, palate. Space between tissue and poorly adapted denture was filled in by this inflammatory growth.

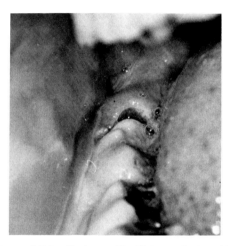

Figure 6.61. Pericoronitis. Note pocket and inflamed tissue distal to a newly erupted third molar.

on the palate and is usually related to ill-fitting dentures and also to poor hygiene. Besides bacteria, fungal (*Candida albicans*) organisms may be found associated with the lesion. The growths are individual masses similar histologically to epulis fissuratum. Treatment consists of removal of the denture after which the condition may subside and new dentures can be made. If the lesions do not subside, surgical excision is followed by the making of new dentures.

Pericoronitis is a common bacterial infection of the gingival tissue, overlying the occlusal of an erupting or partially impacted tooth, usually a third molar. A pocket is created by the flap of tissue (operculum) over the tooth and around the crown (pericoronal) (Fig. 6.61). Food debris can lodge and set up an infection. The ensuing inflammation causes swelling. Often the opposing tooth compounds the problem by adding trauma to the tissue and a cycle of irritation is set in motion. Young adults are mainly affected. There is swelling, extreme pain, some necrosis of marginal gingiva, and foul odor. Depending on host resistance, there can be fever, lymphadenopathy, spread of the infection and pain referred to the ear from the mandibular tooth. Treatment consists of irrigation of the pocket area and frequent rinses with peroxide and water. Antibiotics may be necessary. A gingivectomy or extraction may eventually have to be done as the condition tends to recur.

Specific bacterial infections of the oral cavity are rare. In these instances, the causative organisms are known specifically. The infections in the mouth may be due to bacteria acting locally to produce specific clinical lesions or acting systemically and yielding oral manifestations.

Acute necrotizing ulcerative gingivitis (ANUG, acute necrotizing gingivitis, ulceromembranous gingivitis, Vincent's stomatitis) is the most common specific bacterial infection of the oral cavity. Localized to the gingivae, it is not seen frequently but may be seen in groups. Because it was seen in many military personnel at the same time, in the past it was called trench mouth and was thought to be contagious. On the contrary, it is not contagious. More probably it affects younger individuals such as college students and armed forces personnel because of the physical and emotional stresses common to the group environment. It is also seen in severe debilitation such as with cancer patients. Necrotizing gingivitis is one of those diseases considered to be psychosomatic in origin. Invariably, individuals afflicted with it admit to a stressful environment plus leading a full life with little rest or sleep and with poor nutrition and lack of hygiene. By some mechanisms the tissue resistance is lowered. The content of the oral flora is altered. Organisms usually present in smaller numbers flourish. In this disease a fusospirochetal comlex, a bacillus (*Bacillus fusiformis*) and a spirochete (*Borrelia vincentii* or *Spirochaeta vincentii*) predominates.

Clinically, the manifestations are characteristic (Fig. 6.62). With a rapid onset, the gingiva develop necrotic lesions. These are confined primarily to the marginal gingiva which becomes bright red. The interdental papillae are destroyed and appear scooped out as if cut off. The base of the ulcer is covered with a white slough or membrane-like mass of dead tissue with organisms. This can be wiped off leaving a raw bleeding surface. ANUG can affect one area and spread to several others. It most frequently is seen at the labial of the lower incisors. There is considerable pain, a foul taste, and a fetid odor to the mouth. The teeth feel "wedged" and the gums bleed readily. There can be fever and lymph node swelling with the drainage of infection to the regional lymph nodes.

Treatment consists of several phases. First the acute phase is treated by gross scaling, debridement, mouthwashes, and aspirin for fever. This is followed by other

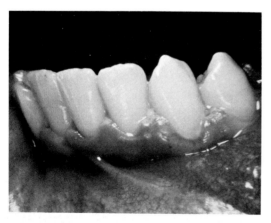

Figure 6.62. Acute necrotizing ulcerative gingivostomatitis (ANUG). Note a progression in severity of involvement from left to right. The interdental papillae become necrotic and disappear. A white pseudomembrane covers the ulcerated gingivae.

appointments with more scaling until healing begins. The patient is advised about proper rest, hygiene, and diet. After the acute phase further periodontal treatment is required. The interdental papillae usually regenerate. If left untreated, the condition will become chronic with repeated acute episodes and severe destruction of the periodontal tissues.

Gangrenous stomatitis or noma is a severe complication of necrotizing stomatitis. Occurring in severely debilitated individuals with protein deficiency or in those being treated with chemotherapy, it is a fulminating infection starting in the mouth and necrotizing through to the facial surfaces. The major problem is the malnutrition and debilitation.

Scarlet fever (scarletina) is a streptococcal disease characterized by a skin rash and a stomatitis. The oral involvement consists of a severe sore throat with a fiery red pharynx and tonsils. The tongue is swollen, red, and coated because of the fever in this disease. The fungiform papillae, also swollen, appear red against the white background resulting in the name, "strawberry tongue." This appearance is not specific to scarlet fever which is now infrequent since the arrival of penicillin. Scarlet fever is caused by a β-hemolytic streptococcus. Oral and throat infections by such bacteria are important to know about because there can be serious postdisease complications. In some individuals there is a sensitization toward the organisms and, after the disease, the body reacts with an immune response that damages its own tissue. Rheumatic fever, kidney disease, meningitis, and subacute bacterial endocarditis may also follow a streptococcal infection.

Syphilis (Lues)

Syphilis is a systemic communicable disease that may have oral lesions. A bacterial infection, it is caused by a spirochete (Treponema pallidum—meaning a pale, twisting thread). A sexually transmitted or venereal disease (VD), the spirochetes are transmitted from one person to another by intimate sexual contact or by close body contact involving the sex organs, mouth, or rectum. The organisms are fragile and cannot live long in light and air; they require warm moist areas for survival. To enter the body, the spirochetes must penetrate mucosa or skin, usually through a wound or area that is not intact. The disease that may ensue has a natural course of three stages with two periods of remission if preventive measures are not taken (Table 6.1).

The primary stage is characterized by the appearance of a chancre (pronounced shank-er). This primary chancre develops at the site of initial inoculation about 2 weeks following intimate contact. Of the lesions, 90% occur on the genitalia and 10% occur in or about the mouth, on the lips, tongue, or palate. The chancre is a hard ulcer that clinically is nonspecific and resembles a traumatic ulcer (Fig. 6.63). It does contain organisms, however. Because of the hard ulcer, cancer is suspected rather than oral syphilis. The ulcer is usually painless and heals spontaneously in weeks. The bacteria spread throughout the blood stream and antibody titers begin to rise. A blood test may be either positive or negative at this time. With the disappearance of the chancre, there is a remission period of months during which time there are no signs or symptoms of disease, except that

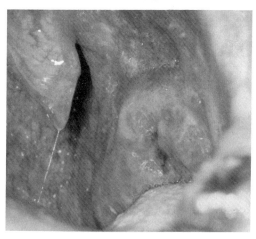

Figure 6.63. Primary syphilitic chancre of left palatine tonsil. The tonsil was very hard, painless, and ulcerated.

Table 6.1.
Natural course of syphilis by stage with indications of oral, systemic, and serologic manifestations

Stages	Incubation Period	Primary Stage	Latent Period	Secondary Stage	Latent Period	Tertiary Stage
Time	3 Weeks, (9–90 days)	3 Weeks	3–6 Weeks	6 Weeks	Months–Years	Years
Oral		Chancre (painless), lip, tongue, tonsil		Mucous patch, papule, rash, condyloma lata		Gumma, atrophic glossitis
Systemic		Adenopathy (painless) ? malaise		Adenopathy malaise syndromes (protean signs)		Cardiovascular disease; Central nervous system disease; other
Serology		−+	++	++++ / +++	+++	+−

the organisms are in the blood and blood tests would be positive. Besides the serologic tests there are antibody tests such as the Treponema immobilization test that is helpful in diagnosing syphilis.

The secondary stage follows the intermission and is characterized by a skin rash, fever, and illness. The skin rash is not distinct and is composed of numerous red macules and papules. These eruptions can occur in the mouth, usually on the palate (Figs. 6.64 and 6.65). The mucous patch is the other oral lesion of secondary syphilis. This is a silvery-white necrotic slough that

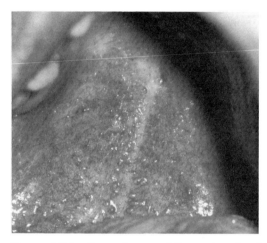

Figure 6.64. Secondary syphilis, oral rash of soft palate similar to herpangina. There was a maculopapular skin rash (Fig. 2.65) including palmar and plantar lesions. Serology was positive.

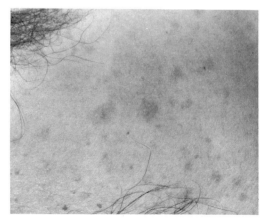

Figure 6.65. Macular skin rash, secondary syphilis.

is highly contagious. It mimics cancer which is what is usually suspected. The lesions of this stage will heal without treatment in several weeks. The blood tests at this stage are definitely positive. With the disappearance of the lesions there is a second period of remission; however, the disease persists. During this time, which can last from many months to several years, the spirochetes settle in various areas of the body and elicit a reaction that in one-third of the patients eventually results in severe damage. Because the oral lesions of primary and secondary syphilis are infectious and contagious, dental personnel should take precautions, such as wearing gloves.

The third stage of syphilis manifests itself primarily with changes in the nervous system and the heart. There is tissue destruction without regeneration, and patients suffer from insanity, loose motor control, and balance. The aorta of the heart in some patients is damaged and causes heart disease. Besides these major findings, there can be oral lesions at this stage. One is atrophic glossitis. The tongue appears smooth, shiny, and bald due to a loss or atrophy of the papillae. A characteristic microscopic picture of syphilis is a perivascular endarteritis. The end arteries become damaged, undergo inflammation, and fail to regenerate causing a loss of the epithelial specialized structures, the papillae. With the normal protection of the papillae being lost, the surface is prone to irritation and white lesions develop (Fig. 6.66). Some of these areas may become cancerous.

The gumma is the other lesion of tertiary syphilis that can involve the oral cavity. They are most frequently seen on the palate. They begin as a nonhealing ulcer that usually is suspected for cancer. There is progressive and extensive replacement of tissue and the destruction may cause a perforation through the soft tissue and bone of the hard palate leaving a permanent opening from the mouth to the floor of the nose (Fig. 6.67).

In the tertiary stage the blood level of antibody usually decreases so that blood

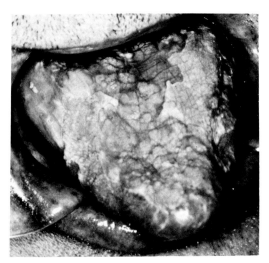

Figure 6.66. Atrophic glossitis of syphilis with leukoplakia.

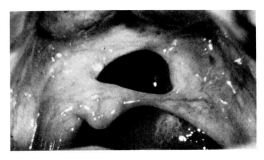

Figure 6.67. Gumma of soft palate, syphilis.

tests can be negative despite the presence of disease. The lesions are not contagious at this stage.

Syphilis can be treated effectively with penicillin. This antibiotic will kill the spirochetes at any stage and stop the disease. However, once the third stage is reached, the damage to nerve, heart, and other tissue will continue on course despite treatment.

Syphilis can be prevented not only by antibiotics and other prophylactic measures but also by conscientious measures and adequate education at all age levels. Syphilis is not simply a bacterial disease. More so, it is a social disease. With better education and responsible social conscience, syphilis could be eliminated.

Congenital or prenatal syphilis is not venereal but is passed on to the fetus by an infected pregnant woman. If the woman is treated within the first 3 months of pregnancy, the fetus will not be affected. After the first trimester the spirochetes pass the placental barrier and infect the fetus. If untreated, most often the disease is fulminating and causes death of the fetus with spontaneous abortion. In other cases, particularly in those fetuses infected later in pregnancy, the baby survives and is born with disease in its secondary or tertiary stages. Numerous organs and tissues can be affected during their development. Visible malformations of having had the disease linger for the life of the child and are called the stigmata of congenital syphilis. These occur in a large percentage, but certainly not in all, of those afflicted with the disease.

Some of these stigmata have been covered under enamel hypoplasia. There can be severe hypoplasia of the primary teeth. In the permanent teeth, Hutchinson's incisors, peglaterals, and mulberry molars can be seen. All are characterized by a decrease in the mesiodistal dimension or a narrowing at the biting surface. Besides these oral lesions, the lesions of tertiary syphilis may ultimately become noted. Sometimes puckering and folds due to scars around the mouth (rhagades) are visible. Bone defects are those manifested by a saddle-shaped nose (depression) and by frontal bossae or bone depressions of the forehead. As a sign of brain damage, the children may be mentally deficient.

Gonorrhea is one of the leading communicable diseases in the United States. Also a venereal disease, the gonococcus organism produces infection with pus. It can be responsible for sterility in women. Women can harbor the disease without signs. During birth the disease can be transmitted to the eyes of the newborn. For this reason silver nitrate drops are applied to the eyes of the newborn for prophylaxis. Gonorrhea is treated with antibiotics but some strains are resistant. However, a vaccination will be available.

The oral lesions of gonorrhea are rare. They are so nonspecific that the suspicion of the disease must be raised by the patient. There may be irregular ulcerations and pharyngitis. Cultures can prove the diagnosis. The oral lesions disappear after antibiotic therapy for the urethral disease. Because the gonococci are anaerobic, there is little chance of transmission of the disease from oral lesions to the dental personnel.

Genital herpes caused by herpes simplex, type 2, is another common sexually transmitted disease. Its pathogenesis is similar to oral herpes (herpes simplex, type 1) in that there may be primary disease and secondary disease caused by reactivation of the dormant virus despite the presence of antibodies. The genital lesions may be transmitted to the oral cavity where vesicles would rupture and a herpetiform ulcer would appear. Likewise, oral herpes may be transmitted to the genitalia.

TUBERCULOSIS

Tuberculosis is an ancient disease caused by the tubercle bacillus, *Mycobacterium tuberculosis*. Whereas in the past it was feared (in 1900, it was the major cause of death) and a disease of social stigma, today it is well controlled because of antibiotics and the centers, originally established primarily to treat it, are treating other diseases. Tuberculosis is primarily a disease affecting the lungs; however, it can involve many other organs. The oral lesions are rare and except where the disease is contacted by unpasteurized milk, the oral lesions are secondary to lesions usually in the lung.

Three strains that can infect man are the human, the bovine (cattle), and the avian (bird). With the advent of pasteurization, it is primarily the human strain that involves man. The bacteria are passed by air through dirt, dust, or continued close contact. They settle in the lung and the body usually reacts with an inflammatory response that effectively seals off the affected area with fibrosis. This can be seen on a chest x-ray and is a sign of the primary contact with the organism. Skin testing may reveal a positive response in many individuals, particularly those living in crowded areas of the city. If the defenses of the body are inadequate on primary contact or with secondary infection, because of an increased sensitivity to the organism, severe damage can take place. The disease can spread in the lung and to the lymph nodes. The organisms are rods with a waxy capsule. By special stain, they appear red or acid-fast. The normal inflammatory response is ineffective and the bacilli cause death of the host cells. Microscopically, granulomas are formed. This is an area of central necrosis where host tissue is destroyed. Macrophages attempt to ingest the bacteria and form a wall around it. Some of them group together to form giant cells called Langhans' giant cells because the nuclei are placed at the periphery of the cell. Special stains may indicate the tubercle bacillus in the cytoplasm of these cells. Also in the granuloma are lymphocytes signifying an immune response and fibroblasts to lay down collagen in an attempt to wall off the response. It presents a specialized picture of chronic inflammation so that microscopic sections can often suggest the presence of tuberculosis. If the host resistance is good, the damage will be localized; otherwise it will spread. The necrosis of tissue is called caseation necrosis because it clinically looks like a white cheese. This eventually will leave a cavity in the lung tissue. If it breaks through blood vessels and a bronchus, there will be a spitting of blood and coughing up of organisms for further spread.

The oral lesions are usually ulcers but may be granulomatous, bumpy, nodular masses. They are nonhealing, persistent ulcers and cancer is usually suspected (Fig. 6.68). A biopsy would reveal that it is not cancer but a granulomatous disease with Langhans' giant cells. If tuberculosis was not known to occur in the patient, further laboratory studies would undoubtedly reveal pulmonary tuberculosis. Tuberculosis may affect lateral neck lymph nodes draining from the oral cavity or a possible jaw lesion. Tuberculosis of a cervical lymph node is called scrofula and would present as a swollen gland by the lower border of the mandible (FIg. 6.69).

Tuberculosis is treated by some isolation, prolonged rest, and the use of appropriate antibiotics combining to effectively reduce

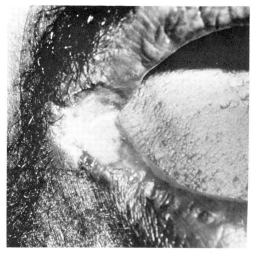

Figure 6.68. A nonhealing ulcer at the commissure of the lips that on biopsy was a tuberculous ulcer. The patient was then found to have active tuberculosis of the lungs.

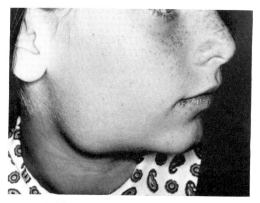

Figure 6.69. Swelling at angle of mandible, firm, movable. On investigation it proved to be a tuberculous lymph node, scrofula.

the morbidity and mortality of this one time major disease.

There are several other granulomatous diseases, some caused by specific organisms, others by foreign materials. Except for foreign body reactions, the other diseases are rare in the oral cavity (histoplasmosis, blastomycosis, sarcoidosis). When they do manifest, there are long-standing lumps, fissures, pebbly, or erythematous areas. There would be suspicion of cancer and the biopsy would show chronic granulomatous disease. Further testing would help to make a definitive diagnosis. The foreign body reaction is the most common granulomatous disease process of the oral cavity.

MUCOCELE

Mucoceles (mucous retention phenomenon) are nodular tumor-like masses caused by some traumatic incident to the mucosa and the minor salivary glands in particular. The oral cavity has numerous clusters of mucous glands with ducts that normally excrete the mucous onto the surface, maintaining a moist atmosphere, accounting for the term mucous membrane. In addition the oral cavity is the site of frequent trauma, which is the leading etiologic factor in many lesions of the mouth. Whereas other lesions created by trauma may have a bacterial component due to secondary infection, mucoceles do not unless surface ulceration occurs.

Mucoceles are common lesions and are diagnosed usually by their clinical appearance. They consist of a soft fluctuant bluish or translucent swelling that can vary in size from a few millimeters to several centimeters. They occur most frequently on the lower lip but may be seen on the buccal mucosa, floor of the mouth, palate, upper lip, and tongue (Figs. 6.70 and 6.71). All age groups are affected, but mucoceles are seen most frequently in children and young adults. The cause is some traumatic injury with the severance of a duct or ducts. The mucus pours into and collects in the adjacent connective tissue rather than the sur-

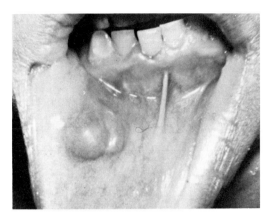

Figure 6.70. Mucocele, inner aspect lower lip in a child.

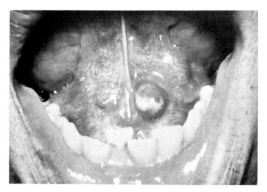

Figure 6.71. Mucocele, floor of mouth at Wharton's duct. Trauma has caused a white lesion on the surface of the soft fluctuant swelling.

A *ranula* is a large mucocele in the lateral aspect of the floor of the mouth arising from a blocked sublingual gland duct. It is called a ranula because of a clinical resemblance to the belly of a frog. The ranula can push the tongue up toward the palate. It is treated surgically either by total or partial removal (marsupialization—removal of cystic contents and healing by secondary intention).

A swelling similar to a mucocele in the floor of the mouth (Fig. 6.71) may be due to a stone within Wharton's duct (sialolithiasis). The patient may complain of pain (not a symptom of mucoceles) and a history that the gland and swelling enlarge while eating. An occlusal radiograph may reveal a round-to-oval opaque mass with concentric laminations (Fig. 6.72). If raised above the surface, it will be a yellow nodule beneath the stretched mucosa. Along with the blockage, there is a retrograde bacterial infection in the gland which will undergo pressure atrophy and fibrosis unless treated. The stone should be surgically removed and the infection treated with antibiotics. Sometimes, the gland has to be removed. Although the submandibular gland and duct are more commonly affected, any gland may be involved, major or minor.

face of the mucosa. The mucus is foreign to the connective tissue, and the body mounts an inflammatory response with granulation tissue to wall if off. A cystlike space filled with mucus is formed, but a mucocele is not a cyst because there is no epithelial lining. Clinically, the fluctuant (fluid motion in a cavity) swelling appears clear like a vesicle if the fluid accumulation is close to the surface epithelium. If the mucus collects deeper in the connective tissue, the swelling appears bluish and may resemble a hemangioma or other blue-black lesion. Often there is a history of swelling, spontaneous rupture, and subsequent swelling. The treatment is adequate surgical removal which should include the associated glands.

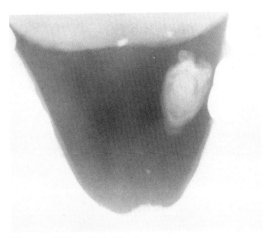

Figure 6.72. Sialolith, floor of mouth, blocking Wharton's duct, radiograph. Submandibular gland was painful and swollen.

MYCOTIC (FUNGAL) INFECTIONS

Fungi are small plants lacking chlorophyll. They are much larger than bacteria and vary in size and shape from round-to-oval cellular masses to long, slender, rodlike hyphae. They are found in plants and animals and generally live a symbiotic parasitic relationship. Fungi occur normally in the oral flora of man. With a lowered resistance or change of the normal floral environment, these fungi can infect man and cause disease. Other fungi, not normally present, may at times also be pathogenic.

Candidiasis (Moniliasis; Thrush)

Candidiasis is a surface infection caused by a yeast-like fungus, *Candida albicans.* The name refers to the appearance of the growth being a glowing white, a characteristic which also places this infection in the category with "white lesions" (see below). The disease occurs essentially in three groups of people. In newborns and babies it is called thrush. The baby presumably contacts the fungus from the vaginal canal during birth. Perhaps the *Candida* flourishes because the oral flora is not well established in newborns and proper balances among organisms have not been achieved as yet. The *Candida* flourishes, appearing as curds of milk on the membrane (Fig. 6.73). Young adults receiving antibiotics or with a lowered resistance are prone to candidiasis. The antibiotic presumably alters the content of the flora and the fungi grows in excess. Other circumstances besides the antibiotic must also be responsible because the incidence of the disease related to the administration of antibiotics is not high. Factors, similar to those seen in necrotizing gingivitis, are frequently present in cases of candidiasis in young adults. The last groups of individuals affected are the debilitated adult patients, most commonly the terminal cancer patients, but also those with long-standing disease. With a lowered resistance, the usually nonpathogenic *Candida* becomes infectious. Of note, it is common in diabetic patients.

Clinically, there are white, irregular, multiple patches that may be seen anywhere on the mucosa. The papular lesions represent the organisms growing in colonies and the necrotic epithelium that they are invading. Characteristically, these white areas can be wiped off which is an aid in diagnosis. The underlying and adjacent mucosa is usually red, after removal of white patches. At times candidiasis may resemble the lesions of lichen planus, another white lesion distinguishable because the white lesions cannot be wiped off (Fig. 6.74). Besides being white, candidiasis may be red and white or just red, as in denture sore mouth. As mentioned in Chapter 4, candidiasis is a causative factor in central papillary atrophy of the tongue.

Candidiasis is treated with antifungal agents such as nystatin or gentian violet. Soothing mouthwashes and sometimes anesthetics may be required for pain and to aid eating.

Other fungal infections of the oral cavity are more rare than candidiasis. They usually are the deep fungal infections. They generally present as nonhealing ulcers suspicious for cancer and are diagnosed by biopsy and other studies, not by clinical appearance.

WHITE LESIONS

White lesions comprise that group of diseases and entities that clinically are char-

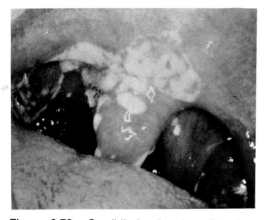

Figure 6.73. Candidiasis, thrush, soft palate and uvula. The white organisms resemble milk curds.

acterized by being white or having some component that is white. The several possibilities of white lesions are listed along with pertinent features in Table 6.2. White lesions are visibly striking because they stand out against the normal pink-red mucosa. Moreover they are important because

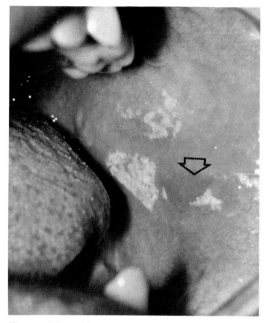

Figure 6.74. Candidiasis, buccal mucosa, in an adult female. The white lesions could be scraped away (*arrow*) and a smear was positive for fungal organisms.

a white lesion may be premalignant or malignant.

The main subgroup of lesions commonly considered when a white lesion is seen or mentioned is that of the keratotic lesions. Among these are leukoplakia, nicotinic stomatitis, and lichen planus. Whereas the latter two clinically can be diagnosed easily because of their characteristic appearances, leukoplakia poses a problem because it may represent one of three separate keratotic conditions.

Leukoplakia is a clinical term indicating the presence of an abnormal white patch that is firmly adherent to the mucosa. It must be defined carefully because it has been used to indicate only premalignancy. In this chapter, it is used as a clinical term only and refers to the lesions that present as white patches or areas. Accepting this, leukoplakia microscopically may be simple hyperkeratosis, hyperkeratosis with dysplasia or actual carcinoma. Of oral carcinomas, 60% present as a white, keratotic lesion or are associated with such lesions. Consequently, white plaques are to be respected and held suspicious until a final diagnosis can be achieved. Further information on oral cancer will be given in Chapter 7.

The white plaques of simple hyperkeratosis and hyperkeratosis with dysplasia are

Table 6.2.
White lesions

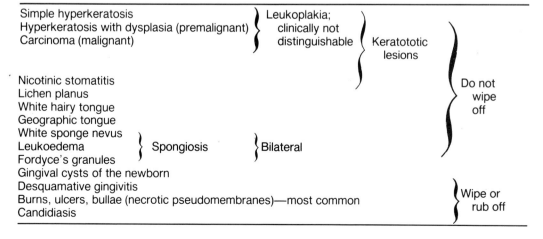

Simple hyperkeratosis	Leukoplakia; clinically not distinguishable	Keratototic lesions	
Hyperkeratosis with dysplasia (premalignant)			
Carcinoma (malignant)			Do not wipe off
Nicotinic stomatitis			
Lichen planus			
White hairy tongue			
Geographic tongue			
White sponge nevus	Spongiosis	Bilateral	
Leukoedema			
Fordyce's granules			
Gingival cysts of the newborn			
Desquamative gingivitis			Wipe or rub off
Burns, ulcers, bullae (necrotic pseudomembranes)—most common			
Candidiasis			

clinically indistinguishable. They appear as white, raised lesions that vary in size, shape, form, and consistency. They may be thin, almost transparent or thick, rough, and skin-like. Often they become stained by tobacco, coffee, tea, or other material. They cannot be scraped away or wiped off with a wooden tongue blade or spatula.

Histologically simple hyperkeratosis is an increase in the surface or corneal layers accounting for the rough texture and white appearance. Depending on the lesion, the keratin layer may be a few layers in thickness or several—to the extent that the keratin or parakeratin layer is thicker than all the other layers of epithelium. By contrast hyperkeratosis with dysplasia contains other cellular changes. Besides a hyperkeratosis, there are the cellular changes of cancer within the epithelium. The only criterion that is lacking to call it cancer is that of invasion into the connective tissue. Because of these changes, hyperkeratosis with dysplasia is considered premalignant. Some dysplasia is irreversible so that at some future time the lesion will become a cancer. The length of time for this ultimate change to take place is not known. Statistically, however, a significantly high percentage of dysplastic lesions do become cancerous if left untreated. Thus this is a very important lesion to diagnose.

These keratotic lesions occur usually in males with a ratio of two males to one female. Usually the patients are about 40 years of age or older. However, depending on the cause, this is not a rigid fact. Generally there are no symptoms and the lesions are found on examination.

There are several causes and factors responsible for hyperkeratosis with and without dysplasia. The most common cause is some local irritation to the mucosa. These include the same factors responsible for trauma to the tissue. Some of these are biting habits, sharp objects such as denture teeth, clasp arms, worn facings on crowns, decayed teeth with sharp enamel edges, and unusual oral habits (Fig. 6.75). These irritate the mucosa, which builds a protection

of keratin or parakeratin against the irritation. Another irritant is smoking which has a drying effect on the mucosa. Cigars and pipes specifically affect the mouth. Cigars may cause a diffuse leukoplakia (Fig. 6.76). The pipe causes discreet lesions on

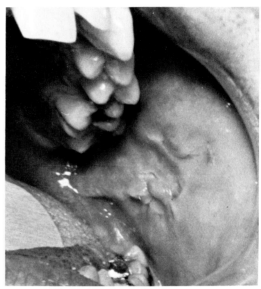

Figure 6.75. Cheek biting. Note many small nodular lesions and areas of leukoplakia.

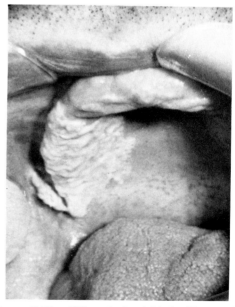

Figure 6.76. Diffuse leukoplakia in 45-year-old male who smokes 15 cigars/day. Biopsies have shown dysplasia.

the lower lip where the stem rests and on the soft palate where the smoke emits from the stem (Figs. 6.77 and 6.78). Cigarettes have their main effect on the lung system. The cilia of the bronchial tree become lost and tars and chemicals build up in the lung. The individual becomes prone to serious diseases such as pneumonia, emphysema, bronchitis, and lung cancer. In addition, the oral mucosa is dried. The drying stimulates a growth of keratin for protection. Holding snuff against the mucosa can also cause similar changes. Nicotinic stomatitis is a clinically distinctive white lesion with simple hyperkeratosis that is specifically

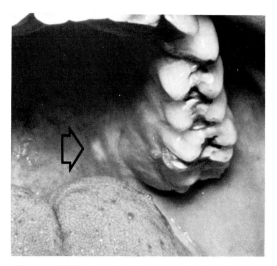

Figure 6.77. Leukoplakia, small discrete area on palate (*arrow*) in a pipe smoker, resulting from smoke and heat emitted at this area.

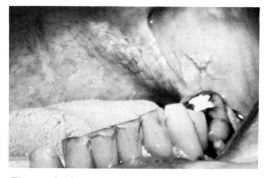

Figure 6.78. Diffuse leukoplakia soft palate, buccal mucosa in a pipe smoker. Biopsy revealed changes of hyperkeratosis.

related to smoking. Some systemic diseases have oral manifestations that allow the mucosa to be sensitive to irritants. Syphilis (atrophic glossitis) and the anemias may result in a smooth bald tongue devoid of the papillae that normally protect the dorsal surface. Frequently leukoplakia can be seen on these tongues, presumably a response to irritants.

The second most common cause of hyperkeratosis is idiopathic because very often no responsible irritant or sustaining factor can be found. Other factors may also play a role in the development of the simple or nonmalignant and premalignant hyperkeratosis. In women, hormonal disturbances may play a role. At menopause with a decrease in estrogen, some women develop areas of leukoplakia. A nutritional deficiency of vitamin A may cause white lesions in rare instances. Heredity probably plays a supporting role since many of the factors mentioned may not cause changes in some individuals as they do in others who may be predisposed by an hereditary pattern.

The treatment for leukoplakia depends on the final microscopic diagnosis. A diligent effort should be made to find a source of irritation since that is the most common cause. If one can be found, the cause should be removed. Simple hyperkeratosis will disappear usually on removal of the cause (Fig. 6.79 and 6.80). If a cause cannot be found or the lesion still persists 2 weeks after an attempt to remove it, a biopsy, either excisional or incisional, should be done. If the microscopic diagnosis is simple hyperkeratosis, continue to search for a cause and remove it. The lesion should disappear. For hyperkeratosis with dysplasia, the lesion should be removed surgically with adequate margins. Any persistent white lesions should be followed and biopsied to determine the microscopic type. Approximately 10% of the leukoplakias excluding carcinomas are dysplastic and 90% are simple hyperkeratotic lesions. However, clinically, they can look alike.

Nicotinic stomatitis is a white, hyperker-

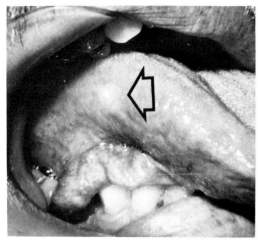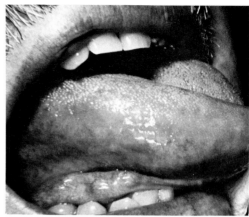

Figure 6.79. *Left,* leukoplakia, middle, lateral border of tongue (*arrow*). Patient rubbed tongue on sharp surfaces on lingual aspect of lower teeth.
Figure 6.80. *Right,* same patient as in Figure 6.79, 1 week after the rough teeth were smoothed. The area of leukoplakia has disappeared.

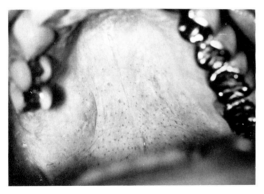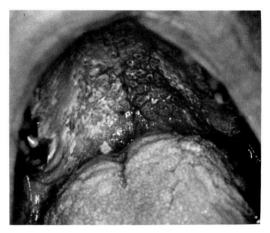

Figure 6.81. Nicotinic stomatitis, hard palate in a cigarette smoker. Note diffuse white background and multiple small areas corresponding to openings at inflamed mucous ducts.

Figure 6.82. Nicotinic stomatitis, hard palate, severe involvement with red and white areas. Several biopsies revealed dysplastic changes.

atotic lesion related as the name implies to the use of tobacco (Fig. 6.81). It is usually seen on the palate in smokers as numerous papules that are white with a central pink, slightly depressed dot. These red areas represent the opening of inflamed and plugged mucous ducts. The white areas represent the hyperkeratosis. These lesions may have a diffuse white background or may be associated with red areas. The palate may have an overall wrinkled effect (Fig. 6.82). A similar response may be seen in snuff holders, usually on the inner aspect of the lower lip or buccal vestibule (Fig. 6.83). In these cases there may be no papules, but the inflamed ductal openings stand out against the whitened background. The treatment includes removal of the smoking or snuff. The lesions are watched carefully to observe their disappearance. If any white lesions persist, a biopsy is necessary to rule out or to confirm premalignancy or malignancy.

Lichen Planus

Lichen planus is the other keratotic lesion that usually has a characteristic clinical appearance so that it can be diagnosed usually without biopsy. Lichen planus is a relatively common disease that affects the oral mucosa as well as the skin and is therefore considered a dermatologic dis-

ease. More often, however, there are oral manifestations without any skin lesions. The oral lesions consist of numerous tiny, white papules arranged in characteristic patterns. The lacelike pattern is most common and usually appears on the buccal mucosa frequently on both sides (Fig. 6.84). The tongue, palate, gingiva (Fig. 6.85) and any other area may be affected. Other patterns are the circular, which on the tongue may mimic geographic tongue, and the plaque-like, which mimics leukoplakia and

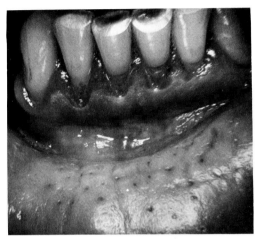

Figure 6.83. Nicotinic stomatitis, lower lip, in a snuff holder. Note leukoplakia and openings of inflamed mucous ducts.

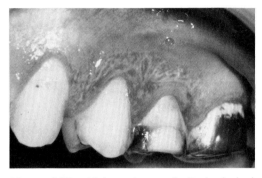

Figure 6.85. Lichen planus of attached gingivae. Note fine, lacelike pattern and red erosive background.

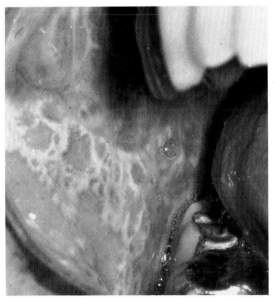
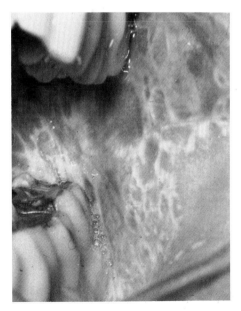

Figure 6.84. Lichen planus, white, keratotic, nonremovable lacelike lesions on both buccal mucosae (two views of same patient on right and left sides).

must be distinguished by biopsy (Fig. 6.86). The oral lesions usually are asymptomatic and are detected on routine oral examination. However, there is an erosive form of lichen planus that may cause discomfort. In these instances, characteristic lesions are usually seen at the edge of the erosive areas. The diagnosis is usually made by the clinical appearance. The coexistence of purple-violet papules on the flexor surfaces of the skin, chest, or genitalia may also be helpful toward diagnosis. In those cases where the clinical appearance is not characteristic and the lesions appear as a leukoplakia, biopsy is very helpful because lichen planus has a specific histologic appearance. Besides the hyperkeratotic surface, there is degeneration at the basement membrane area and a characteristic lymphocytic infiltrate congregated immediately adjacent to the epithelium. This pattern allows the pathologist to distinguish the disease as lichen planus.

Lichen planus is probably a psychosomatic disease because there is usually some specific emotional event relating to the start of or the exacerbation of the disease. The actual cause is unknown. An immune disturbance is suspected. And the disease is notable among diabetics. The treatment in most cases consists merely of diagnosis. The lesions may last for weeks, usually months or even years. They eventually will disappear with or without medication. Topical steroids are very effective. Sympto-

matic treatment is required in erosive disease. Lichen planus is an innocuous disease. Patients can be reassured that it is not cancer and is not serious.

Other White Lesions

White hairy tongue is a harmless condition in which the filiform papillae fail to shed normally and become elongated. The causes vary and include heavy smoking, antibiotic therapy, poor hygiene, emotional tension and idiopathic factors. The midposterior dorsal surface is most often affected; however, the lateral borders may be involved. The "hairs" may pick up stains from bacteria, smoking, tea, coffee, or candies. Treatment consists of removal of the cause. Brushing the tongue aids in promoting removal.

Geographic tongue has white lesions at the periphery of the atrophic reddened areas. These desquamative and hyperkeratotic areas often assume circular patterns similar to lichen planus and traumatic glossitis from denture irritation. Characteristically, however, the atrophic areas heal in one area and appear in others—helping to distinguish this harmless condition from other white lesions.

White sponge nevus is a hereditary condition which presents as white, soft folds of tissue bilaterally on the buccal mucosa mainly, but also on the tongue and floor of the mouth. The white appearance is due to the spongiosis or fluid in the cells. It is usually diagnosed clinically on the basis of being bilateral and with the aid of a familial pattern. Biopsy would confirm the spongiosis and rule out hyperkeratosis.

Leukoedema also appears bilaterally on the buccal mucosa. There is a spongiosis of the spinous cells which yields a silvery, shiny white lesion with some wrinkles (Fig. 6.87). The linea alba is usually accentuated. Hyperkeratosis can be ruled out clinically by stretching the mucosa. When this is done, the white lesion "disappears" (Fig. 6.88). Leukoedema is commonly seen in black patients. The cause is unknown. Some correlation exists between the sever-

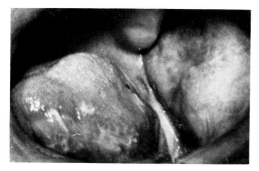

Figure 6.86.   Lichen planus, buccal musoca and tongue. Areas of leukoplakia occur along with a lacelike, linear pattern.

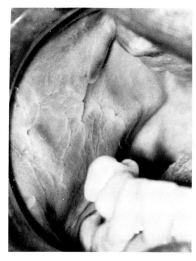 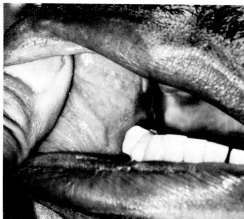

Figure 6.87. *Left*, leukoedema, buccal mucosa. Note folded, white spongy appearance.
Figure 6.88. *Right*, leukoedema, same as in Figure 6.87. When tissue is stretched, the white disappears.

ity of leukoedema and poorer oral hygiene. Leukoedema is essentially a normal condition and must be differentiated from the more serious white lesions.

Fordyce's granules (Fig. 1.10, 1.14, and 4.13) are usually seen bilaterally on the buccal mucosa and on the lips. They may be noted as white or yellow-white submucosal clusters that appear more prominent when the tissue is stretched taut. They are normal sebaceous glands without hair follicles and occur so frequently they are considered normal. Sometimes a large cluster on the buccal mucosa concerns a cancerophobic patient. The patient should be reassured they are not cancerous. There is no treatment.

Gingival cysts of the newborn, commonly called Epstein's pearls, are mentioned here only because they are white lesions. They appear on the gingival pads in infants, not adults (Fig. 6.89). These keratin cysts disappear spontaneously. Sometimes they mimic an erupting tooth.

The following group of white lesions can be distinguished readily from the keratotic variety because they can be wiped away with a wooden tongue blade or metal spatula.

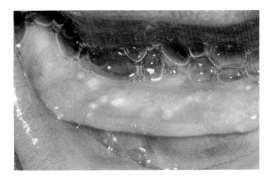

Figure 6.89. Gingival cysts of the newborn (Epstein's pearls) on gum pad of a 6-week-old boy.

Desquamative gingivitis is a condition seen primarily in women about the age of menopause. It may present as a burning sensation affecting the gingiva. There are erosive or red areas associated with white areas representing the desquamating epithelium that can be wiped away exposing more reddened areas. Desquamative gingivitis is actually a clinical term because the condition can be seen in other diseases such as allergies and dermatologic-oral diseases.

Three diseases that can present with desquamative gingivitis are erosive lichen planus, mucous membrane pemiphigoid, and pemphigus.

Pemphigus, like lichen planus, is a dermatologic disease with oral manifestations, but unlike lichen planus, it is quite serious because it is fatal if left untreated. Moreover, the oral lesions are often present before the skin lesions and afford the observer an opportunity to refer the patient for early diagnosis and treatment. It affects older patients of Jewish or Mediterranean origin. Pemphigus is an autoimmune disease affecting spinous cells. Large vesicles can form anywhere in the mouth and soon rupture. The necrotic epithelium is white and accounts for the white lesion against a red background (Fig. 6.90). The lesions may be seen on routine examination or are reported to have been present for some time. As nonhealing ulcers and erosions, they should be suspicious. Biopsy is important because pemphigus has a specific microscopic picture. Besides intense chronic inflammation, there is an intraepithelial vesiculation and acantholysis. This can be contrasted to other bullous and erosive diseases which have subepithelial vesicles. Pemphigus can be debilitating and fatal

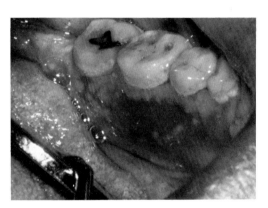

Figure 6.90. Pemphigus vulgaris, presenting as a desquamative gingivitis. Biopsy, smear and other tests were positive.

because the lesions on the skin ulcerate and expose a large surface area with loss of fluids similar to third degree burns. It can be effectively treated by immunotherapy.

Mucous membrane pemphigoid affects older women with blisters on the gingivae, primarily, and other areas such as the palate. An autoimmune disease, it shows subepithelial blistering with antigen-antibody complexes in the basement membrane zone. The skin may be involved as well as the conjunctiva, in which case scarring may lead to blindness. Thus, steroid therapy is required.

Another dermatologic-oral disease with sloughing white blisters is erythema multiforme. An acute condition, it is characterized by lip lesions that crust on the skin side. Within the mouth, the lesions are white from necrotic epithelium and red. On the skin, there may be a rash in many forms (multiforme), including a lesion with concentric rings (target lesion). The genitalia may be involved. When the disease is severe and the conjunctiva are involved, it is called Stevens-Johnson syndrome. The cause is unknown but usually there is an allergen or hypersensitivity state. If discovered, the allergen should be removed otherwise there will be recurrences. The use of steroids is effective even though the disease is self-limiting and spontaneously regresses with supportive therapy.

Burns, ulcers and other lesions with a white, necrotic surface or pseudomembrane comprise the most common group of white lesions. The white part of the lesion wipes off and leaves a raw surface. This fact, plus additional history and clinical features, will usually distinsuish them from the keratotic lesions. On the other hand, there are serious diseases among this group. Oral cancer may present as an ulcer.

CHAPTER 7

Benign and Malignant Conditions

NEOPLASIA

An introduction to neoplasia was presented in Chapter 2. This section will offer further clarification and some details of a most complex aspect of pathology.

The term neoplasia refers to a new growth of tissue. If growth of tissue relating to developmental and inflammatory hyperplasia is excluded, there are essentially two categories of neoplasia—benign and malignant. Any tissue of the body that is capable of dividing is capable of developing a neoplasia, a basic tissue response to various stimuli, in which the growth control mechanism is defective. The resulting growth may show cellular changes with little, if any, variation in morphology or behavior from the normal. This is one extreme of a large spectrum of changes that may occur. At the other extreme, the cells may not resemble or behave like the cells of origin, in which case, they are called poorly differentiated. Thus, new growth may be hyperplastic; if the cause is removed, the growth of normal tissue stops. The growth may be abnormal: with little variation from the normal, it is benign; with marked variation, it is malignant.

Benign growths are those that are not malignant or highly injurious. Their cells resemble those of the tissue of origin. They are usually slow growing, encroaching on normal tissue as they expand. With expansion, a connective tissue capsule develops around them and the growth remains localized. Usually the removal of them is straightforward, recovery is quite favorable, and they do not recur. As a growth, however, they create a mass that must be distinguished from a malignant growth (Fig. 7.1).

Malignant growths, by contrast, are highly injurious. Their cells are atypical and deviate markedly from the cells of origin. The nuclei are usually enlarged and occupy more of the cell than normal. The cell size is often enlarged and there may be giant cell formation. The cells may lose all resemblance to the normal cells and cannot be recognized (anaplasia). Numerous mitotic figures account for the rapid growth. Some of these mitoses may be abnormal. The cells lose contact with one another and the arrangement of cells is disorderly. They grow by infiltration and invasion into the surrounding normal tissue. No capsule is formed; there is no localization. The hallmark of a malignant growth is its capacity to spread, i.e. metastasize. The growth may spread directly by extension, by sending cells into the lymphatic or vascular channels. The cells may grow at a distant site but generally do so at sites of preference, usually related to a rich blood supply. Thus, the lung is a frequent site for metastasis. Breast and prostatic malignancies metastasize to bones. Consequently, a radiolucency in the jaw can be due to a metastasis. Because of metastasis, the treatment of a malignancy is not straightforward and recovery is not always favorable. The prognosis depends upon the extent of size and spread of tumor (staging) at the time of discovery. The greater the spread, the worse the prognosis. Recurrences are not unusual. A patient with one malignancy is likely to develop another. Consequently, malignancies are followed closely and are measured in terms of 5- or 10-year cure rates. Some of the distinguishing features between benign and malignant growths are given in Table 7.1.

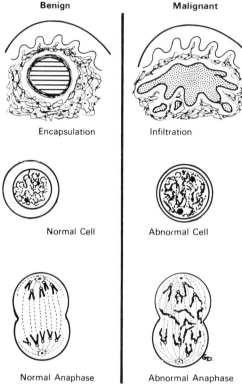

Figure 7.1. Diagram comparing features of benign and malignant tumors.

The naming of neoplasms is generally done by utilizing the name of the tissue of origin. Table 7.2 offers a classification of some of the benign and malignant neoplasms. Most benign neoplasms are designated by adding the suffix "-oma" after the name of the tissue of origin. For example, a benign neoplasm composed of fibrous connective tissue is called a fibroma. If two or more tissues comprise the neoplasm, the terms are combined and the tissue of greater prominence appears last as in neurofibroma. However, although the suffix "-oma" connotes a tumor or neoplasm, there are exceptions that exist. A granuloma is not a neoplasm although it may present as a swelling or tumor. A lymphoma is not a benign neoplasm of lymphocytes but is, in fact, malignant. *Cancer* is the general term used for a malignant neoplasm. Cancers of epithelial origin are called *carcinomas*; cancers of mesodermal or connective tissue origin are called *sarcomas*. Exceptions are the lymphoma and the melanoma for which the prefix malignant offers no confusion. The leukemias are malignancies of the blood-forming cells.

The effect of the neoplasia on the patient depends on the site or location, on the type of neoplasm, and on the individual patient. Benign growths create masses that are usually investigated to determine the presence of a malignancy. They usually are not fatal but can be if they expand and cause pres-

Table 7.1.
Distinguishing features between types of a neoplastic mass

Neoplasia	Benign	Malignant
Clinical	Mass	Mass
	Capsule (localized)	No capsule (infiltrating)
	Slow growth	Rapid growth
	No metastases	*Metastases*
	Usually not fatal	Fatal if untreated
Microscopic	Cells, typical; normal	Cells, atypical; abnormal size, shapes
	Regular arrangement	Loss of regular arrangement
	Few mitoses	Many mitoses, often abnormal
	Normal nucleus	Large nucleus

Table 7.2.
Classification of neoplasms

Cell or Tissue of Origin	Benign	Malignant (*Cancer*)
1. *Epithelium*		*Carcinoma*
Surface		
Squamous	Papilloma	Squamous cell carcinoma
		Verrucous carcinoma
		Basal cell carcinoma
Respiratory	Papilloma	Nasopharyngeal carcinoma
	Inverted papilloma	
Glandular	Adenoma	Adenocarcinoma
Salivary duct	Pleomorphic adenoma	Malignant pleomorphic adenoma
Pigment cells	Pigmented nevus	Melanoma (malignant melanoma)
Tooth	Ameloblastoma	Malignant ameloblastoma
2. *Connective tissue*		*Sarcoma*
Fibrous	Fibroma	Fibrosarcoma
Adipose	Lipoma	Liposarcoma
Cartilage	Chondroma	Chondrosarcoma
Bone	Osteoma	Osteosarcoma
Neural nerve	Neuroma	Neurosarcoma
Schwann cell	Schwannoma	Malignant schwannoma
combined	(Neurilemoma)	Malignant neurilemoma
	Neurofibroma	Neurofibrosarcoma
Vascular	Angioma	Angiosarcoma
Blood vessels	Hemangioma	Hemangiosarcoma
Lymph vessels	Lymphangioma	Lymphangiosarcoma
	Cystic hygroma	
Pericytes	Hemangiopericytoma	Malignant hemangiopericytoma
Granular cells	Granular cell tumor	Alveolar soft part sarcoma
Blood forming		Lymphoma, leukemia, myeloma
Tooth	Odontogenic fibroma	
Muscle		
Smooth	Leiomyoma	Leiomyosarcoma
Skeletal	Rhabdomyoma	Rhabdomyosarcoma
Histiocyte	Fibrous histiocytoma	Malignant fibrous histiocytoma
3. *Mixed*—epithelial and connective tissue		
Tooth	Odontoma	
	Ameloblastic fibroma	Ameloblastic fibrosarcoma

sure on vital parts. Some benign tumors of glandular origin may produce secretions or hormones that can severely affect the patient. An adenoma of the parathyroid gland can cause an excess of hormone so that calcium is mobilized from bones and osteolytic and radiolucent lesions are seen in bones. These may appear in the jaws as a manifestation of the systemic disease called von Recklinghausen's disease of bone. The removal of the parathyroid adenoma cures the bone lesions. Other effects of benign growths may arise from complications such as hemorrhage or infections that can arise because of their presence.

Similar effects can arise from malignant growths. Cancer and benign growths may present in many ways. On body surfaces which can be readily examined, the growth may be a "lump" or a sore that fails to heal. On internal organs, it may present as pain. Cancer, however, is usually painless until its later stages. There may be bleeding or some other sign depending on the organ affected. An example is hoarseness in cancer of the larynx. The most important physiologic effect, though, is cachexia, a wasting resulting in weakness and weight loss. This may directly cause deaths, but the primary danger is because it predisposes the patient to infections. A prime cause of death in cancer patients is infection (pneumonia) and suicide. Another factor governing the effect of the growth is the state of the resistance of the individual patient. Resistance is a complex and poorly understood physiologic phenomenon. Contributing to it is immunity and its role in counteracting or containing malignancies.

The cause of cancer in humans is unknown. It appears that there are many factors that may act in concert with one another to produce an irreversible change in the nucleus of a cell so that given a chance to proliferate it will grow uncontrollably. Some of these factors that are recognized as having a probable effect in the cause of cancer are: viruses, chemicals, hormones, family susceptibility, physical agents, immunity, aging, diet, and sex.

There are recognized viruses that cause cancer in animals. In man, a strain of herpes virus, Epstein-Barr, is responsible for the Burkitt's lymphoma, a malignancy of the maxilla affecting children in certain parts of Africa.

Chemicals that can cause cancer are called carcinogens. Polycyclic hydrocarbons painted or implanted in animals produce cancer. Similar compounds have been associated with cancer in man. Smoke from cigarettes contains many carcinogens. The tars and chemicals adhere to the lung tissue. With a decreased resistance, familial tendency toward cancer, and the carcinogens, a lung cancer or bronchiogenic carcinoma may develop. Cigarette smoking is directly related to the incidence of lung cancer.

An imbalance of hormones can be related to cancer. An excess of hormones may lead to hyperplasia of cells at the target organ. Such a stimulation could eventually result in neoplasia. Cancer of the breast has been related to the hormone estrogen as well as to a familial susceptibility toward the disease. Certain families are more prone to certain types of cancers. Given a predisposing set of factors for cancer, individuals in these families can react in a similar pattern resulting in neoplastic disease.

Immunity plays a significant role. If the immune response is decreased, there is a greater chance of inducing neoplasia and existing neoplasia is enhanced. Interestingly, immunity decreases with age. With age there is a greater susceptibility to cancer. With some exception, cancer is a disease of older age. One can ponder that those individuals dying of lung cancer related to smoking at age 55 probably would have died of the same disease at 75. The smoking and other factors may have altered the immune response so that the development of the neoplasia occurred years earlier.

Various physical agents are related to cancer production. Ionizing radiation such as x-rays in chronic exposures can cause cancer. Diagnostic radiation may affect the unborn fetus who later in life may get leukemia. Radiation from the sun can be a factor in skin cancer. This is particularly true of light-skinned individuals who are exposed either by occupation or by choice to sunlight. Likewise, chronic mechanical trauma or irritation can contribute to neoplasia. Irritation constantly applied to an area coupled with other factors can produce a neoplastic growth.

In the development of a neoplasia, there is a neoplastic change imposed on a cell in the mitotic phase. If a differentiated cell is the target, a benign tumor will result. If an undifferentiated or stem cell is the target, a malignant tumor will result. Three steps are recognized: initiation, promotion, and progression. In initiation there is the exposure to the mitotic cell by a carcinogen. A single exposure is enough. But other factors, promoting agents such as chemicals (esters) and irritation, are required to promote the changed cell to proliferate. Other factors, not defined, allow the progression of this group of cells to the development of a malignancy. In the epithelium, there is a recognizable premalignant phase called epithelial dysplasia. Dysplasia may progress to include all of the epithelium, called carcinoma in situ. The cells have all of the attributes of cancer cells but there is no invasion into the underlying tissue. Once the cells invade and permeate the connective tissue then the growth of changed cells is called a carcinoma. Then the cancer cells can spread. Epithelial cancers generally spread first to lymph nodes and secondly to the blood stream. Sarcomas tend to spread by blood vessel, the multistep process of metastasis may follow. If the cells survive they are transported to a distant organ, arrest in and penetrate the capillary. Again exposed to further body defenses, the cells may survive and proliferate setting up a cancer in the secondary site (metastasis) (Fig. 7.2).

The treatment for neoplasia varies. Benign neoplasms are cured usually by simple surgical removal. They generally do not recur. Malignant neoplasms are treated by surgery, radiation, chemotherapy, or a combination of these. Some malignancies behave similar to benign growths and are easily cured. Others are not easily cured and may offer a grave prognosis depending on the type of cellular characteristics. Because there is a spectrum of cellular changes in cancers, these can be graded by the pathologist. Generally a low grade malignancy, the cells of which tend to resemble the tissue of origin, has a better prognosis than a high grade malignancy. Some cancers may be inoperable and incurable, in which case palliative and supportive therapy is used to relieve pain and discomfort. Even when an apparent cure is accomplished, patients with cancer must be watched closely because of the possibility of metastases being present and not dis-

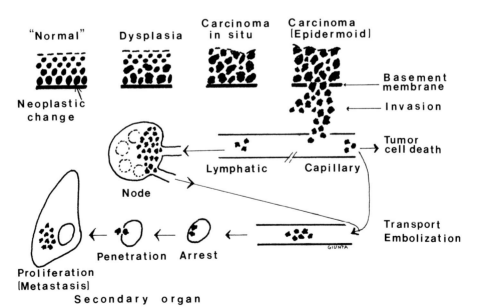

Figure 7.2. The development of a squamous cell carcinoma and a metastasis. Features are: invasion; spread via lymph and blood vessels; and steps progressing to a secondary neoplasm (metastasis).

cernible, because recurrences are frequent and because they are prone to more than one primary cancer.

Cancer is indeed a malicious disease. It is the second leading cause of death in the United States. Because of this impact, extensive efforts continue both clinically and at the research level to unravel the secrets of neoplasia, a common response of the body to the various stimuli about it resulting in hundreds of diseases (cancers).

BENIGN TUMORS OF THE ORAL CAVITY

Of the neoplasms, the benign tumors are much more common than the malignant and comprise a large percentage of the most common oral lesions observed and biopsied in dental practices. They can arise from any tissue of the oral cavity, including that within the bone. Usually they present as a swelling or nodular mass projecting outward from the mucosa. They may be attached to the mucosa by a narrow stalk or pedicle, in which case they are called pedunculated. If the base of the lesion is broad or wide the attachment is called sessile. In many instances the dignosis is strongly suspected clinically, and because the treatment is usually surgical removal, the tissue is submitted for confirmation by microscopic analysis. In other circumstances the diagnosis is not definite and an incisional or excisional biopsy is done for definitive diagnosis. Any nodular mass or swelling of tissue should be suspected as being a neoplasm, inflammatory hyperplasia, or developmental hyperplasia, and followed-up until adequate diagnosis and care are instituted.

Fibroma (Irritation Fibroma)

The fibroma is a nodular mass composed of dense fibrous connective tissue. It is one of the most common lesions of the oral cavity and may occur in any location, although the buccal mucosa, tongue, lower lip and gingiva are sites most affected. The fibroma appears as a pale pink to white, raised, smooth surfaced, firm mass which may be pedunculated or sessile and can vary in size from a few millimeters to centimeters (Fig. 7.3). Because it is associated with some irritation or trauma, it is often referred to as an irritation fibroma inferring that it is not a true benign tumor. Rather, it may reflect the end stage of a chronic imflammatory response, but the dense bundles of collagen, of which it is composed, are indistinguishable from those of a true fibroma. In addition, some inflammatory cells are invariably present. Cheek biting may lead to a fibroma on the buccal mucosa. Other habits such as rubbing a rough area with the tongue may likewise result in a lesion called a fibroma. Fibromas are readily diagnosed clinically. Treatment is simply surgical excision and microscopic examination. They may recur if the irritant is not removed.

Other lesions are composed of the same dense, firm tissue as the fibroma. Several of these affect the gingivae or the mucosa of the alveolar ridge. Because the area affected is diffuse, the term fibromatosis is used to indicate that the large mass of tissue resembles the fibroma. Fibromatosis of the gingivae has been referred to under developmental lesions (Chapter 4). In this familial disease the gingivae are enlarged and tumor-like but microscopically they are composed of dense fibrous connective tissue. Dilantin hyperplasia of the gingivae is a similar condition, but the cause is the administration of the drug dilantin for epilepsy. In some patients receiving the drug, the gingivae enlarge with a fibromatosis (Fig. 7.4). Transplant organ recipients on immunosuppressants may get a similar fibrotic reaction of the gingivae. Removal of the drug or gingivectomies are the treatment. Fibromatosis unrelated to a familial tendency or to dilantin is frequently seen in some patients in the maxillary tuberosity areas. These areas may be so enlarged that they favor periodontal disease or, in edentulous patients, they will interfere with fabrication of dentures. Surgery is the treatment. A fibroma on the gingiva may be

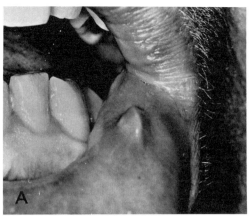
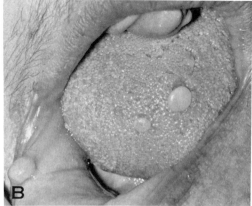

Figure 7.3. *A*, Fibroma, sessile base, lower lip. Patient had habit of biting lip at this site. *B*, Multiple fibromas, tongue and buccal mucosa.

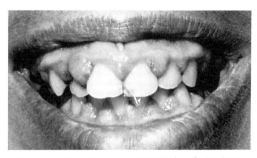

Figure 7.4. Dilantin hyperplasia of gingivae.

large or small and, because of its location at the interdental papilla, may be termed a fibroid epulis. They are like fibromas elsewhere but must be distinguished from the peripheral giant cell granuloma, the pyogenic granuloma, and the hemangioma.

Angiomas are benign tumors composed of vascular channels. If the channels contain red blood cells, the tumor is called a hemangioma. If the vascular spaces are filled with lymph fluid, the tumor is a lymphangioma. The hemangioma is the most common benign tumor of the oral mucosa. Because of its cellular nature, it is often diagnosed but not removed with such frequency as the fibroma. Moreover, the hemangioma, unrelated to irritation, is considered a true tumor. Some pathologists refer to it as a hamartoma, meaning that there was an overabundance of normal tis-

sue formed, in this case blood-filled channels.

Hemangiomas are often congenital and may be present at birth or appear in childhood. They tend to enlarge slowly and often regress in size at puberty. The hemangioma appears as a red, blue-red, or purplish lesion that may be flat or raised and can vary widely in size (Fig. 7.5). The color may blanch on pressure and a pulsing often can be felt in the smaller lesions. Hemangiomas occur in all sites of the oral cavity—the tongue, buccal mucosa, and lips being common sites. Sometimes the lesions may be extensive. Half or all of the tongue may be involved and create a macroglossia (Fig. 7.6). In lymphangiomas of the tongue there are usually small projections with clear fluid yielding a pebbly appearance rather than a smooth surface. The treatment for hemangiomas varies with the individual circumstances. They may be left alone and observed. Precautionary measures should be taken against irritating or injurious factors. They may regress at puberty. Small lesions may be excised easily. Others may be injected with sclerosing solutions that promote scarring.

Hemangiomas are seen on the face and neck. Flat, large, red-purple areas, usually present from birth are called port-wine hemangiomas or stains. These cause cosmetic

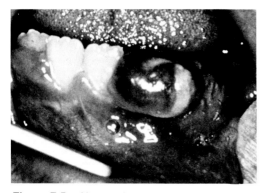

Figure 7.5. Hemangioma of gingiva (epulis) in a 6-month-old male. Lesion has been traumatized and has necrotic areas (white) on surface.

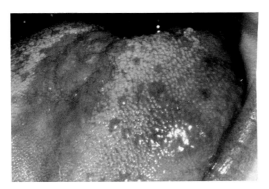

Figure 7.6. Hemangioma, left side of tongue, in a 9-year-old who also has central papillary atrophy (median rhomboid glossitis).

most frequently on the ventral surface of the tongue and on the posterolateral surface near the lateral lingual tonsils. They appear as prominent deep purple or blue-black lesions. No treatment is required.

Capillary hemorrhage may cause red or purple macules called petechiae to appear on the mucosa. The soft palate is a common site (Fig. 7.9). Causes vary from the common cold, other viral diseases, to trauma or

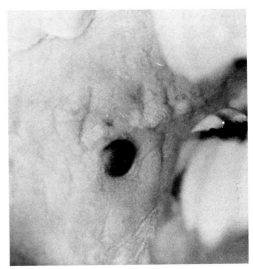

Figure 7.7. Hematoma or blood blister, buccal mucosa due to cheek bite.

difficulties but may be successfully covered since surgery and radiation are contraindicated.

There are other vascular lesions to be considered which are not tumors. A *hematoma* is a blood blister. It is a collection of blood beneath the mucosa. Usually deep purple, the lesion may be flat or raised. Secondary to trauma, the buccal mucosa and lower lip are common sites (Fig. 7.7). Patients on anticoagulants such as dicumarol are prone to bruising and may cause large hematomas (Fig. 7.8). The collection of blood cells is gradually resorbed and the lesions disappear without intervention.

Vascular channels can dilate and become tortuous. This phenomenon of varicosities is common in aging individuals. It is seen

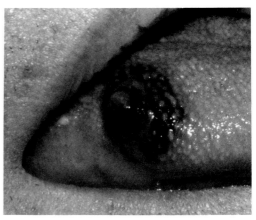

Figure 7.8. Hematoma, lateral tongue in male patient on coumadin because of kidney dialysis treatment. Patient bit tongue and caused this bruise.

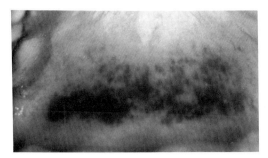

Figure 7.9. Multiple punctate, purplish, petechiae and ecchymosis of soft palate. Usually due to trauma, this can be a sign of a bleeding problem.

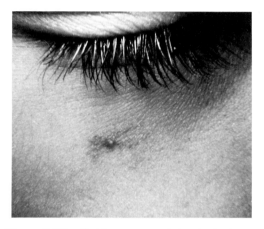

Figure 7.10. Spider nevus or telangiectasia on face below eye. This red lesion blanches upon pressure.

bleeding disorders. The spots turn blue or yellow prior to their disappearance.

Telangiectasias are small, red macules or papules formed by dilated capillaries. They may be round or have spider-like appearances (Fig. 7.10). They are common on the face, particularly the lips and nose. The causes vary and there is a hereditary form. As with other vascular lesions, precautions against trauma and irritation should be taken.

The lymphangioma is a rare tumor of the oral cavity. It may occur singularly or be a component of a hemangioma. It is usually congenital and may cause severe enlargement of the affected part. The tongue is a usual site, and it may present as a macroglossia in an infant. Treatment is similar to that of the hemangioma.

Neuromas are rare lesions of the oral cavity. Because of the functioning nerve tissue, these nodular masses are usually painful. Some trauma is generally associated with their occurrence. Treatment is surgical removal.

A more common lesion is the neurofibroma, a benign tumor of combined origin in which the basic fibroma has nerve elements. Neurofibroma produces nodular masses that may be large and softer in consistency than the firmer fibromas (Fig. 7.11). Like the fibroma, it may be multiple. However, when neurofibromas occur, they may be part of a systemic disease called multiple hereditary neurofibromatosis (von Recklinghausen's disease). Affected individuals have numerous neurofibromas on the face, the body, in the mouth, and in internal organs. In addition, they have pigmented, raised nodular lesions and several large brown macules called cafe-au-lait spots, like birthmarks, scattered over the body. It is important to diagnose and to watch these people because some of the neurofibromas may become sarcomas later in life.

Lipoma

The lipoma is a rare benign tumor derived from adipose tissue or fat wherever it

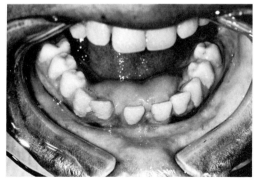

Figure 7.11. Neurofibroma, lingual gingiva. Note separation of teeth due to pressure of tumor.

occurs in the oral cavity. The buccal mucosa and retromolar areas are common sites. The lesions appear as nodular masses which may be yellowish in color because of the fat. They tend to be soft in consistency. They are composed of normal fat cells. Treatment is simple excision.

Papilloma

The papilloma is a common tumor derived from squamous epithelium. It is a white lesion because of the keratotic surface. Nodular, it is usually characterized by a rough surface with a pebbly texture or with numerous small, slender, thick hairlike projections emanating from a pedunculated or sessile based mass (Fig. 7.12). The size is generally confined, ranging from millimeters to about 1 centimeter. The papilloma can occur anywhere and is seen on the gingiva, tongue, uvula, floor of mouth, and lips. Similar appearing lesions are seen on the skin of the face and fingers. They are called verucca or warts because some are caused by the human wart virus (papovavirus). Some appear as a result of irritation. Papillomas are benign, however, large lesions may resemble a verrucous carcinoma. The treatment is complete surgical removal.

Pleomorphic Adenoma (Benign Mixed Tumor of Salivary Glands)

The pleomorphic adenoma is a benign tumor of salivary gland origin. It is derived from ductal epithelial cells and has a varied pattern (pleomorphic). These lesions are not common. Most of them occur as swelling emanating from the parotid gland where they comprise 75% of all the tumors at that site. Thus, a swelling at the angle of the mandible, in a middle-aged person, near the ear is probably a pleomorphic adenoma (Fig. 7.13). However, it cannot be distinguished from a malignant lesion or other tumors that can arise from the parotid. It is a swelling that must be investigated. The pleomorphic adenoma is also the most common intraoral salivary gland tumor. Its usual location is the palate where it presents as a smooth surfaced swelling resembling a fibroma (Fig. 7.14). The upper lip is the next most common site. Treatment is wide surgical removal since they tend to recur.

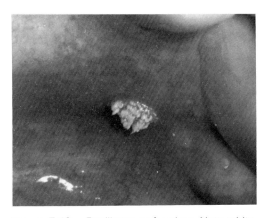

Figure 7.12. Papilloma, soft palate. Note white, keratotic, finger-like projections and a flat (sessile) base. This is wartlike.

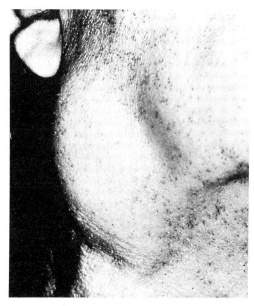

Figure 7.13. Pleomorphic adenoma, parotid. Large swelling at angle of mandible had been present and increasing in size over many years.

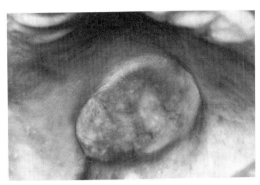

Figure 7.14. Salivary gland neoplasm, pleomorphic adenoma, hard and soft palate. This swelling was covered by a denture.

Odontogenic Tumors

Odontogenic tumors are those derived from cells that normally would form a tooth or part of a tooth. Most are benign. Very rarely, one is malignant.

ODONTOMA

The odontoma is the most common odontogenic tumor, occurring usually before the age of 20. It is generally noted on radiographic examination. There is usually a circumscribed area with a central radiopaque mass composed of numerous toothlike objects or dense irregular masses and spicules surrounded by a narrow radiolucent zone (Fig. 7.15). It occupies the space of a missing tooth or represents a developmental defect of a supernumerary tooth. Sometimes the jaw may be expanded or teeth may be separated. The odontoma may interfere with the eruption of a tooth. The radiographic picture is characteristic. Conservative surgical removal is the treatment. The mass is composed of all the elements that form a tooth—pulp, dentin, cementum, and enamel—and is, therefore, mixed in origin. They may be either regularly arranged, like small teeth, or irregularly arranged (Figs. 7.16–7.18).

An odontogenic fibroma or pulpoma is derived from the connective tissue part of the tooth-forming organ. It probably represents the aborted development of a tooth in its early stages and is characterized by the proliferation of pulplike or fibrous tissue. Radiographically, there would be a radiolucent lesion.

AMELOBLASTOMA

The ameloblastoma is a benign tumor, derived from dental lamina, enamel organ cells or cyst epithelium, and composed of epithelial cells resembling those of the enamel-forming organ of a tooth. It is histologically benign but can be locally aggressive, invading and destroying bone. It usually occurs at age 30 or older but can appear at any age. Its common location is the posterior part of the mandible. As it slowly increases in size the jaw enlarges causing disfigurement (Fig. 7.19). Radiographically, there is a radiolucent cystlike appearance. It may mimic a solitary cyst but usually has a multicystic or compartmentalized appearance as if several soap bubbles were joined

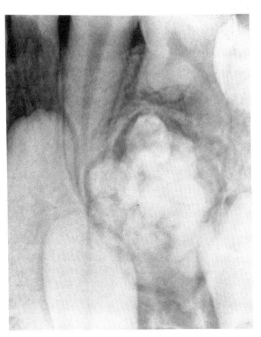

Figure 7.15. Composite odontoma, mandible, in 8-year-old. Multiple radiopaque toothlike masses with surrounding radiolucency. This was interfering with eruption of the premolar.

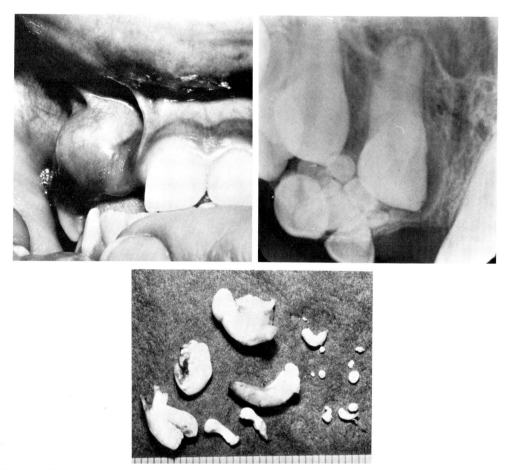

Figure 7.16. *Top left*, odontoma, 11-year-old female. Presents as a hard swelling alveolar mucosa. Note missing teeth.
Figure 7.17. *Top right*, radiograph of odontoma, multiple small radiopaque objects. Also note unerupted permanent teeth.
Figure 7.18. *Bottom*, multiple irregularly shaped, tooth-like objects removed on surgery.

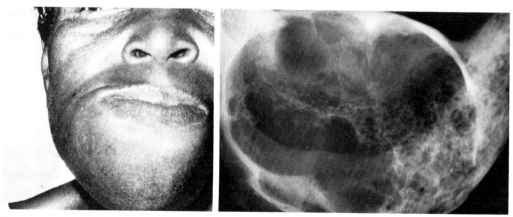

Figure 7.19. *Left*, ameloblastoma, mandible. Note disfigurement and enlargement of jaw.
Figure 7.20. *Right*, ameloblastoma, multiocular or soap-bubble radiolucencies and thin radiopaque trabeculations.

together (Fig. 7.20). There can be extensive destruction of the bone. Nonencapsulated islands of ameloblastic cells and stellate reticulum infiltrate and permeate the marrow spaces of the bone. Consequently, treatment consists of wide excision and, depending on the case, may involve removing a segment of or half of the jaw. They may also arise from the wall of a dentigerous cyst usually associated with an impacted lower third molar (Fig. 7.21), in which case, they behave less aggressively.

Two other odontogenic tumors may manifest as dentigerous cysts radiographically overlying an impacted tooth. Both occur in younger people than the ameloblastoma, usually in the first or second decades. The adenomatoid odontogenic tumor is a nonaggressive encapsulated lesion of ameloblastic cells with duct formations. Usually occurring in females about a maxillary, impacted canine, it is easily removed and does not recur. The other tumor, derived from both ameloblastic cells and dental papilla tissues (a mixed tumor), is the ameloblastic fibroma. Frequently seen in youngsters in the posterior mandible, this tumor is encapsulated, removes easily from the bone but may recur.

CEMENTOMA

The true cementoma (cementoblastoma) is a rare odontogenic tumor composed of cementum with an active and aggressive

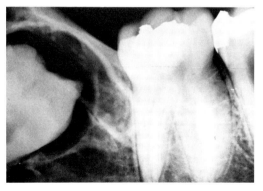

Figure 7.21. Ameloblastoma arising in dentigerous cyst.

growth pattern. Usually it is noted on a radiograph as a dense, opaque mass surrounding and attached to the cementum of the root end of the tooth. In its early stages it could resemble hypercementosis. They may occur in the absence of a tooth, in which case they resemble enostoses or other opaque bone lesions. Due to progressive growth and intimate attachment, the tooth and tumor must be surgically removed together.

NONTUMOR BONE LESIONS

Periapical cemental dysplasia, commonly called cementoma, is not a tumor of odontogenic origin composed of cementum. As partly described in Chapter 5, it is a condition of unknown etiology, occurring in tooth-bearing bone that, in its early stage, may resemble periapical inflammatory disease. There are three stages that can be recognized in the development of this condition, the radiographic appearance reflecting what is happening microscopically within the bone. The earliest stage is a radiolucent lesion; fibrous tissue replaces the bone. With time, calcified masses form within the fibrous tissue giving a combined radiolucent and radiopaque (ground glass) lesion. The final stage is one in which there is more bone or cementum than fibrous tissue resulting in a mostly radiopaque or cotton-wool appearance. Mandibular anterior region is most often affected. The teeth test vital. There is no jaw enlargement and the cementoma requires follow-up by radiographs and biopsy only to rule out other entities.

Fibrous dysplasia of bone is a disease of young people of unknown cause. There is a replacement of bone with fibrous tissue containing varying amounts of abnormal bone. These can affect long bones and those of the skull and jaws. The jaws may be enlarged and teeth may migrate or separate (Fig. 7.22). The radiographic appearance and histologic stages are similar to cemental dysplasia (Fig. 7.23). However, the sites vary, with the maxilla and posterior mandible being preferred sites. The bone lesions

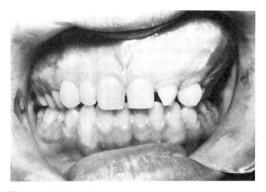

Figure 7.22. Fibrous dysplasia of maxilla in a 20-year-old male. Note enlarged left maxilla and separated teeth. This was a firm mass.

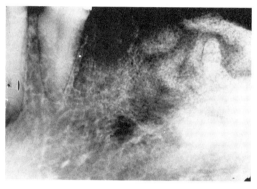

Figure 7.23. Radiograph showing changes in a confirmed case of fibrous dysplasia. There is a combination of radiolucent and radiopaque areas including a ground glass and cotton-wool appearance.

are diffuse and not well defined. The treatment consists of diagnosis, and possible surgery for cosmetic reasons only.

Condensing osteitis previously mentioned in Chapter 5 may resemble end stage cemental dysplasia. A sequelae or sign of a chronic pulpitis, the radiopaque lesion is most often noted surrounding the root or roots of a lower molar tooth that usually has a large restoration or decay (Fig. 7.24). Biopsies show some chronic inflammation about dense bone spicules.

Eosinophilic granuloma is a bone disease that can mimic a tumor or periodontal disease. It is characterized by proliferating macrophages plus eosinophils which infil-

trate the bone causing a punched-out, cystic radiolucency or a radiolucency around the roots of teeth looking like advanced periodontal disease. The teeth may be mobile, an unusual sign because eosinophilic granuloma occurs in young people. Biopsy is needed to prove the diagnosis. Treatment is surgical excision or low dose radiation. The disease may recur and act aggressively.

ORAL CANCER

Oral cancer is the most important disease to detect in the oral cavity because it is a killer and because it occurs with a relatively high frequency. It comprises approximately 5% of all malignancies. About 15,000–20,000 will be detected in 1 year. However, only 7,000–10,000 of those detected will be cured and living in 5 years. The cure rate for intraoral cancer is worse than that for cancer of the uterus. This comparison is made because the oral cavity is more accessible for visible examination than the uterus. Oral cancer is detectable in its early stages so that it can be found and cured. Greater efforts at early detection, patient awareness and motivation would change the present bleak statistics.

The etiology of oral cancer is unknown.

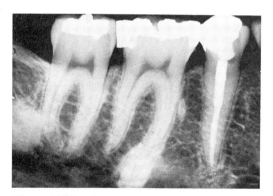

Figure 7.24. Radiograph with multiple lesions. Opacity near mesial root of first molar at middle third is consistent with a retained primary root tip. Opacity at apical end of mesial root is consistent with condensing osteitis. Opacity distal to second molar is consistent with periapical fibrous dysplasia or enostosis. Also note overhanging margin of restoration on first molar on distal and calculus on mesial.

However, there are several factors associated with an increased incidence of oral cancer.

Tobacco use is a prime factor. In the mouth there is a drying effect which causes irritation and promotes the buildup of keratin. Cigars, pipes, and snuff are particularly harsh on the oral mucosa. Cigarettes also have an effect but primarily involve the lungs. Tobacco also contains carcinogens that may act locally in susceptible individuals. Oral cancer occurs in significantly more smokers than nonsmokers.

Alcoholic consumption on a regular, habitual basis is another factor. Few cases of oral cancer appear in individuals who do not drink alcoholic beverages. Often smoking and drinking are combined habits.

Chronic irritation is another prominent factor. Oral cancer is associated with keratotic lesions in about 60% of the cases. This implicates chronic irritation. Sources for irritation are ill-fitting dentures, sharp edges on partial dentures, jagged restorations or rotten teeth, and any oral habit that inflicts damage.

Other factors that are responsible for predisposition to irritating factors are syphilis and anemias. Atrophic glossitis of tertiary syphilis and certain anemias result in a bald tongue which is prone to irritation and leukoplakia. A percentage of such patients will get cancer of the tongue.

Poor oral hygiene is a condition associated with oral cancer. Not infrequently, a typical oral cancer patient is one who smokes heavily, drinks heavily, and disregards oral hygeiene. Such patients are not motivated to visit the offices of dentists or physicians. Therein lies the challenge for early detection. On the other hand, oral cancer does occur in mouths of those who do not drink or smoke and who are motivated toward good health habits.

Oral cancer affects males more than females in a ratio of 4:1. This statistic may change since the female is smoking as much as the male is now. The age of occurrence is 40 or older; however, younger individuals are not immune.

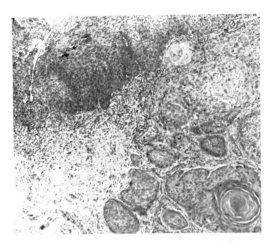

Figure 7.25. Squamous cell (epidermoid) carcinoma invading connective tissue at right. Adjacent surface epithelium at *left* is dysplastic. Tumor is forming keratin (*lower right corner*).

Of all oral cancer, 95% is squamous cell or epidermoid carcinoma derived from the epithelium of oral mucosa (Fig. 7.25). Because they are mucosal, changes can be seen. The high risk areas in order of frequency are the lower lip, lateral border of tongue, floor of mouth, buccal mucosa, palate, tonsils, and gingiva. Oral cancer can be separated into lip cancer and intraoral cancer because of the differences in prognosis.

Lip cancer occurs primarily in males past 50 years of age. It affects the lower lip usually in the lateral aspects (Fig. 7.26). The lesions are usually painless, small keratotic or white areas with erosion and ulceration. There may be crusting at the skin surface. They may feel hard. With time they grow into large masses and present as ulcerative swellings of the lip. These are usually well differentiated, low grade lesions which generally do not metastasize. They offer a good prognosis with 5-year survival rates of 90–95%. Tobacco and actinic radiation are associative factors. Actinic radiation from the sun affects light-complexioned individuals who work out-of-doors and produces changes in the skin and lower lip. The skin appears flushed and burned with prominent telangiectasis over the cheeks, nose, and lower face. The lower

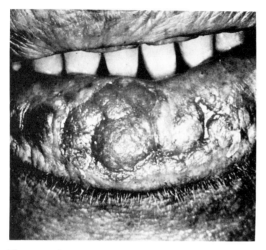

Figure 7.26. Epidermoid carcinoma, lower lip, diffuse involvement.

until late stages are reached. A patient may be unaware of even a large lesion. The early changes to be searched for are ulcers, white areas, smooth or rough areas, red and white pebbly areas, red velvety areas, a swelling, or a papillary mass (Figs. 7.28 and 7.29). The late changes may be firm ulcers, masses, pain, bleeding, difficulty in swallowing, lymphadenopathy (metastases), weakness, and weight loss. There is no specific description of oral cancer. It is detected by a systematic routine of careful and deliberate oral examination and by having a high index of suspicion. A nonhealing ulcer or red pebbly lesion and particularly a red and white lesion, that persists beyond 2 weeks should be considered

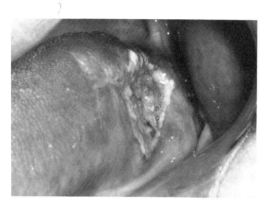

Figure 7.27. Epidermoid carcinoma, posteriolateral border of tongue in a 60-year-old smoker and drinker. There is a large ulcer as well as adjacent red and white lesion.

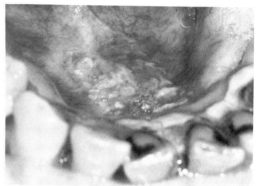

Figure 7.28. Epidermoid carcinoma, floor of mouth and lingual ridge. This was a speckled red and white slightly raised painless lesion.

lip appears blanched and dry, smooth and swollen, and often has small white plaques. This is called solar cheilosis and is considered to predispose to a small number of lip cancers. Treatment usually consists of a stripping of the vermilion border or wedge resections and plastic surgery for favorable esthetic and functional results.

Intraoral cancer comprises all areas other than the lip. The tongue is the most common site. The areas of the tongue of high risk are the posterolateral surfaces and the ventral surface, not in the dorsum or midline (Fig. 7.27). Intraoral cancer is painless

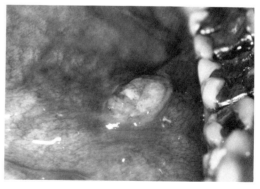

Figure 7.29. Epidermoid carcinoma, floor of mouth, in a 43-year-old female smoker and ex-drinker. This small size and early discovery means a better prognosis.

cancer until proven otherwise. Keratotic lesions must be biopsied to rule out premalignancy and malignancy, since a large percentage of oral cancer is associated with white lesions. Erythroplakia, a red plaque not considered part of a known disease must be biopsied since most are dysplastic or cancerous. Only a constant awareness of the possibility that any lesion not otherwise accounted for may be cancer will the early cancer be detected.

Oral cancer is diagnosed by biopsy. The oral biopsy is accurate in diagnosing oral cancer on the first biopsy in nearly 100% of the cases. Oral cytology may be valuable and can detect cells from the mouth. However, it is accurate in only 85% of the cases and should not be used instead of the biopsy. Any patient with a suspicious lesion should be referred to a dentist or physician for biopsy and follow-up.

Intraoral cancer contrasts with lip cancer. The type of cancer tends to be of a higher grade and tends more to metastasize to the lymph nodes of the neck. The more posterior the tumor, the more the tumor has spread at time of diagnosis and the worse the prognosis (Fig. 7.30). The prognosis is only fair since there is a 5-year survival rate of 50%. The survival rates reflect treatment of these patients. This rate increases markedly, though, if the original lesions are less than 1 cm and if there are no metastases, stressing again the importance of early detection. The treatment consists of surgery, radiation therapy, a combination of the two, or chemotherapy where only palliative therapy is useful. Precautions must be taken when radiotherapy is used in the head and neck. Since it induces xerostomia, the teeth should get treatments to prevent radiation caries (Fig. 7.31). Treatment is usually directed by a team of cancer specialists. If the lesion is small, limited surgery or radiation alone can effect a cure with limited disfigure-

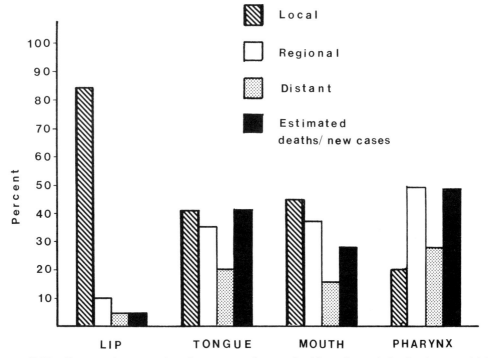

Figure 7.30. Bar graph comparing the extent of spread with estimated deaths (prognosis) for cancers of the lip, tongue, mouth, and pharynx. As the cancer is more posterior, the spread at initial discovery is greater and the prognosis is worse.

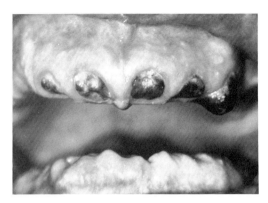

Figure 7.31. Radiation caries secondary to xerostomia in an oral cancer patient treated with radiation only. Unfortunately, poor hygiene and lack of fluoride therapy resulted in this preventable loss.

ment. In larger lesions and those with metastases, extensive, mutilating surgery may be required. Plastic surgery and prosthetic appliances may be required to ameliorate the resulting defects. All oral cancer patients are followed closely because they may have a second primary tumor or a recurrence.

Intraoral malignancies other than the squamous cell carcinoma exist but are rare. The most common is the intraoral salivary gland malignancy. The most usual site is the palate where the lesion presents as a firm, painless, growing mass whose growth may be slow or fast. They may invade the bone. Treatment is surgical and prognosis is poor.

Other malignancies are those of connective tissue origin. These sarcomas are extremely rare, rapidly growing nodular masses that may ulcerate. Melanomas are black lesions of malignant nevus cells. They rarely occur intraorally but the site of preference is the palate or gingiva.

More frequent than the mesenchymal lesions are the metastatic bone lesions. These are metastases to the jaw, usually the mandible, from primary malignancies elsewhere, like the breast, prostate, thyroid, lung or colon. They present as radiolucencies, may or may not produce pain, and may cause loosening of the teeth.

Regarding lesions in the bone, either primary or secondary, there are significant symptoms. If a patient complains of a tingling (paresthesia) of the lip or any numbness, pain, or swelling and it is not associated with a dental origin, a malignancy of bone should be suspected and further investigation is required.

Extraoral cancers of the face and neck are usually visible on examination. (Figs 1.1 and 1.2). The most common cancer of skin is the basal cell carcinoma, commonly seen on the upper face and neck. It is a tumor rising from and composed of the basal cells of the epithelium of the skin. It is found in older individuals, generally fair skinned, who are exposed to the sun. The lesions occur anywhere—upper lip, nose, ear, and neck. Usually they are small, rounded, raised or only slightly raised, red or scaly lesions often with a central depressed area of ulceration. It is a "sore" that fails to heal. Characteristically, it is slow growing, localized, spreads by local extension, and rarely if ever metastasizes. It is easy to cure with conservative surgery or radiation. If left untreated, or if discovered as a large lesion, extensive infiltration and destruction can occur and the treatment is more radical and less likely to cure. When diagnosed and treated early, there is usually a 95% cure rate.

PIGMENTATIONS

Pigmentations are of two types, endogenous and exogenous. Those pigments produced by the body are endogenous. Those introduced from the environment are exogenous. Some of the pigmentations seen in the oral cavity are listed in Table 7.3 which separates them into categories of diffuse and focal. Diffuse or spread out pigmentation usually signifies that there is a systemic problem elsewhere in the body. Such a manifestation of systemic disease is seen in Peutz-Jeghers syndrome. The oral signs are numerous brown macules or spots of melanin about the lips and perhaps in the mouth. The systemic problem is inherited multiple polyps or growths in the in-

Table 7.3.
Pigmentations

Distribution	Endogenous	Exogenous
Diffuse—spread out	Metabolic—systemic disease	Industrial
	Melanin spots	
	Peutz-Jeghers syndrome	Lead, silver, etc.
	Adrenal insufficiency	
	Bilirubin	
	Jaundice—black teeth	
Focal—localized	Normal melanin	Amalgam tatoo—common
	Hemosiderin	Foreign bodies
	Blood product	(pencils, etc.)
	Black teeth	
	Melanotic macule	Tetracycline—yellow-brown
	Nevus	
	rare in mouth	
	Melanoma	

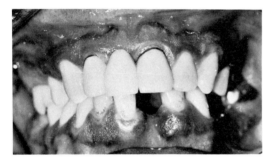

Figure 7.32. Normal melanin pigmentation, gingivae.

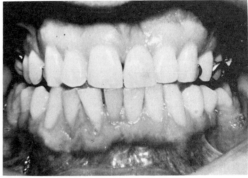

Figure 7.33. Intrinsic staining, lower incisor. Gray color due to bleeding into dentinal tubules. Patient had history of being hit by a baseball bat. Also note the supernumerary lower incisor (five incisors).

testine. These have the potential of causing obstruction and rarely become malignant. Patients with diffuse pigmentation should be suspected of having a systemic problem and should be referred to a physician.

Certain occupations and some medical therapy can introduce heavy metals into the body. These settle out in many organs, one of which can be the mouth, particularly along the marginal gingiva.

The more common pigmented lesions of the oral cavity are those that are focal or localized, not diffuse. Normal melanin pigment is seen frequently, particularly on the attached gingivae (Fig. 7.32). Usually physiologic melanin is symmetrical but a single patch may occur. History may help differentiate it from a melanotic macule. There

is no clinical significance to physiologic melanin except to recognize it as normal. Hemosiderin and bilirubin are pigments of blood breakdown. The hematoma is a collection of blood that presents as a blue-black round lesion usually on the buccal mucosa. Petechiae are macules of hemorrhage that are blue-black at first and then change to a yellowish color as the blood products are broken down and disappear. Bleeding into the dentinal tubules leaves red blood cells that break down and cause a staining so that the tooth appears darkened. (Fig. 7.33). This is commonly

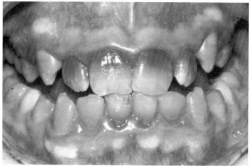

Figure 7.34. Staining of teeth due to excess bilirubin. This resembles tetracycline staining and dentinogenesis imperfecta.

melanotic macule (freckle) is a brown spot caused by melanin in the basal cell layer (Fig. 7.35). A nevus is a flat or slightly raised benign tumor mass with nevus cells and melanin in the connective tissue. A melanoma is a malignant nevus, appears black, and occurs rarely in the mouth, its common site being the palate and alveolar mucosa.

The other focal pigmentations are exogenous. The most common is from the embedding of amalgam particles in the con-

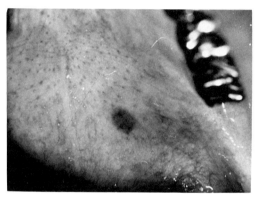

Figure 7.35. A melanotic macule on the soft palate. This could be simple melanin pigmentation, a nevus, or a melanoma; also note the nicotinic stomatitis.

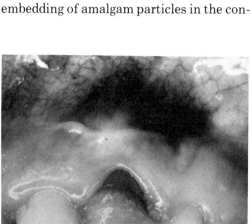

Figure 7.36. Amalgam tattoo, labial sulcus due to retrograde amalgam filling of cuspid which had a dead pulp and is stained due to hemosiderin in dentinal tubules.

seen in anterior teeth that have been traumatized. A dark tooth should be investigated for pulpal or periapical pathology. Black or gray-black teeth may be due to medications and a systemic condition causing a breakdown of blood into bilirubin pigment causing jaundice. The pigment remains in the dentinal tubules and stains the teeth black (Fig. 7.34). This had been seen in children born of mothers with an Rh incompatibility with the baby (erythroblastosis fetalis). The newborn can be transfused with blood and saved; however, black or gray-black primary teeth remain as a reminder of the episode of jaundice.

Other focal lesions are associated with melanin but are rare to the oral cavity. A

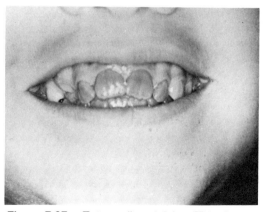

Figure 7.37. Tetracycline staining. This change is permanent but bleaching or bonding may help eliminate the surface discoloration.

nective tissue of the mucosa. These "amalgam tattoos" appear as small, well defined, blue-black lesions, occurring in association with the alveolar ridge. The particles of amalgam may show as radiopacities on a radiograph. They may result from the placement of retrograde root canal fillings, appearing in the mucobuccal fold (Fig. 7.36). They occur in older individuals who have usually had extensive dental treatment. Often they are noted on the alveolar ridge after extraction of teeth. In the floor of the mouth, they may resemble melanin pigmentations. Amalgam tattoos are so common that they should always be considered when a black lesion is noted. Other diagnostic considerations should include the mucocele, hemangioma, and melanin pigmentations.

Other foreign materials may cause pigmented lesions. Many individuals habitually introduce lead pencils into the mouth. Graphite from the pencil can be forced into the mucosa and leave a dark, black circumscribed macule resembling the amalgam tattoo (Fig. 6.13). A careful history will aid the differentiation.

The antibiotic tetracycline may cause permanent intrinsic staining of either the primary or permanent teeth. If tetracycline is given over an extended period of time to the mother during pregnancy or to the infant, the teeth developing at that time will be stained from a mild yellow to an unsightly yellow-brown or grey (Fig. 7.37). The change is permanent. The permanent teeth may need bleaching, bonding or crowns to improve the esthetics.

CHAPTER 8

Oral Manifestations of Systemic Diseases

Numerous examples of oral manifestations of systemic diseases have been mentioned in other sections of this chapter. Viral diseases, tuberculosis, syphilis, lichen planus, pemphigus, and pigmentations are some examples. The oral cavity is commonly involved in many systemic diseases. Sometimes the resultant lesion is easily categorized and specific so that the disease entity is recognized, e.g. lichen planus. Other times the oral lesion is nonspecific. The lesion(s) may be common for several disease states that must be distinguished by means other than the clinical lesion itself. Thus, the oral manifestation may be gingivitis, glossitis, cheilosis, stomatitis, hemorrhage, infection, ulceration, pigmentation, changes in tooth eruption patterns, enlargement of bone, or other general disease states. One or more of these conditions may coexist and, along with other body signs and symptoms, reflect a generalized, systemic disease rather than merely a localized, oral disease. A few more examples will be noted in this section.

Angular cheilosis refers to a fissuring or ulceration of the lips specifically at the angles of the mouth. The condition may be painful, annoying and long lasting. There are several causes. A common localized etiologic factor is the loss of vertical dimension of the occlusion in partially or totally edentulous individuals. Without the appropriate stops, the mandible overcloses toward the maxilla. The lips are forced against one another and appear grooved inward at the angle of the mouth (Fig. 8.1). Saliva leaks out and creates a moist environment harboring microorganisms. Eventually the tissue breaks down and ulcerates. In this case, the vertical dimension can be restored by appropriate dental prosthetic appliances. Other causes of angular cheilosis are excessive salivation, with drooling and infection with *Candida albicans* in which case the name of *perleche* is synonymous with cheilosis. Nutritional deficiencies, anemias and allergy may also be etiologic factors in angular cheilosis.

True nutritional deficiencies are rare in the United States although they may be found in deprived individuals or in those who practice "diet" fads. Vitamin B complex rather than an individual vitamin B deficiency may result in angular cheilosis as one of its signs (Fig. 8.2). Usually coupled with the cheilosis and generally regarded as the main oral sign is an atrophic or "bald" tongue (Fig. 8.3). There is atrophy and loss of the filiform and fungiform papillae. The tongue appears smooth; is prone to irritation; and often becomes red, swollen, and painful.

Atrophic glossitis is also seen in anemic states. In the anemias there is a decreased amount of oxygen available from the red blood cells to the tissues. The tongue is sensitive to such changes in its nutritional state and responds with a loss of papillae resulting in a smooth tongue (Figs. 8.4 and 8.5). Blood tests must be done to accurately diagnose the type of anemia. Pernicious anemia is a hereditary disease wherein the patient lacks an instrinsic factor necessary to absorb vitamin B_{12}. After diagnosis and treatment with monthly injections of vi-

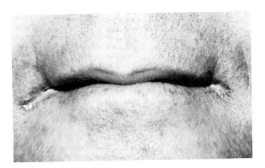

Figure 8.1. Angular cheilosis due to loss of vertical dimension in a full denture wearer.

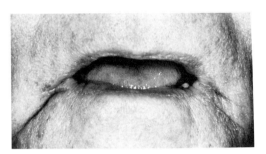

Figure 8.2. Angular cheilosis associated with vitamin B complex deficiency as well as loss of vertical dimension.

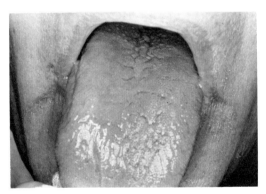

Figure 8.3. Smooth balding tongue and angular cheilosis associated with vitamin B complex deficiency. Same patient as in figure 8.2.

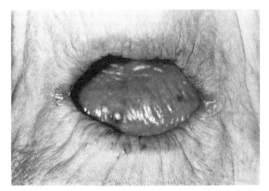

Figure 8.4. Angular cheilosis and pallor of the lips associated with iron deficiency anemia in a 76-year-old female with Plummer-Vinson syndrome.

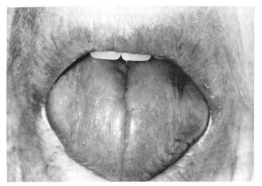

Figure 8.5. Smooth bald tongue associated with iron deficiency anemia. Same patient as in figure 8.4.

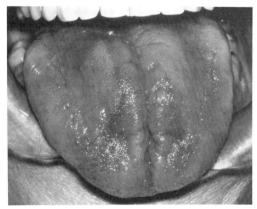

Figure 8.6. Smooth patchy red tongue due to vitamin B_{12} deficiency secondary to pernicious anemia.

tamin B_{12}, the mucosa returns to normal (Figs. 8.6 and 8.7). It should be recalled that the endarteritis of syphilis produces atrophic glossitis in the tertiary stage of the disease. The loss of papillae may occur gradually leaving patchy areas that may

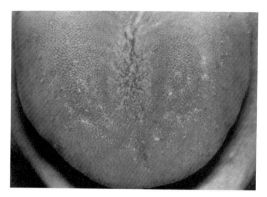

Figure 8.7. Normal appearing tongue of patient in Figure 8.6 after treatment with injection of vitamin B$_{12}$, showing regeneration of lingual papillae.

mimic traumatic glossitis or geographic tongue. Tongues with atrophic glossitis are susceptible to the development of leukoplakia and therefore may also have white patches over the smooth red surface.

Another sign of anemia may be the pallor of the skin and mucosa. The lips may be white with a bluish tint in addition to the cheilosis and glossitis.

Gingivitis, with red, boggy, swollen, bleeding gingivae, may be a sign of systemic disease. Systemic disease may alter the response of the tissue to local factors or it may, in itself, cause a hyperplastic response. The resulting clinical picture is recognized only as a gingivitis. Generally, patients with gingivitis of local cause will heal dramatically after a scaling and curettage. If after such treatment(s), a patient fails to heal or the lesions on the gingiva persist, some systemic disease or component should be considered. An imbalance of sex hormones at puberty, pregnancy, menstruation, or via oral contraceptive agents have been associated with gingival inflammation. Diabetic patients are prone to severe periodontal problems and may also have an increased tendency toward pulpal and periapical inflammation. Oral dryness, burning, and tenderness are common complaints in a patient who has or may have diabetes mellitus. Bleeding and hyperplastic gingivae may be a sign of vitamin C

deficiency (scurvy), although this would be very rare now. Leukemia may predispose the gingiva to a hyperplasia. The enlarged tissue may be due to inflammation or an infiltration of the leukemic cells. Sometimes the gingival lesions may be the first sign of this malignant disease. Generally, acute monocytic leukemia is the type with gingival lesions (Fig. 8.8). However, other signs such as lymphadenopathy, bleeding, and petechiae and ulceration may also occur.

Gingivitis and bleeding, in particular, may be caused by a bleeding or hemorrhagic disorder. There may be bleeding in the mucosa as well so that hematomas develop. Multiple deep blue lesions may occur. Eosinophilic granuloma is a disease in which cells infiltrate tissue, particularly bone. In the jaw it causes a resorption of bone surrounding molar teeth in particular. On the radiograph there is a radiolucency showing severe localized destruction resembling a cyst, but the teeth appear to be floating with no support. The teeth may be quite mobile. The mucosa may be involved resulting in a gingivitis. This localized gingival inflammation plus the radiographic picture often will be the first signs of the disease. Thus, gingivitis may be a sign of systemic difficulty in a patient.

Macroglossia may be a sign of systemic disturbances. A large tongue is seen in several disorders. Acromegaly, a hormonal disturbance in which there is usually an adenoma of the pituitary gland with an in-

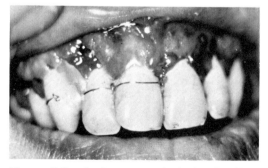

Figure 8.8. Acute monocytic leukemia. Note gingival swelling, areas of erosions, and bleeding.

crease in growth hormone, results in enlargement of the skull, mandible, hands, and feet. Connective tissue hyperplasia occurs, and the lip and tongue enlarge dramatically. A decrease in thyrotropic hormone, hypothyroidism may result in cretinism in the newborn or myxedema in juveniles and adults. Of many manifestations, one is a large tongue caused by the edema in the tissue. Because of pressure against the teeth, the tongue may have a scalloped appearance along the lateral borders. Features other than the enlarged tongue exist in these conditions, but the tongue will be the striking feature during the oral examination.

Macroglossia occurs in other conditions and has been referred to in other chapters of this module. Because the condition is striking and because several categories of disease are represented in the finding of macroglossia, its causes are interesting to review and offer an overview of general pathology utilizing a single condition. Essentially we are referring to a diffuse enlargement of the tongue, causes of which may be congenital, acquired, or idiopathic (Table 8.1).

Congenital macroglossia may be seen in patients with mongolism. This is a spontaneous or hereditary genetic defect with several manifestations, one being a large tongue. Hemangiomas and lymphangiomas are developmental benign tumors that may affect the entire tongue (angiomatosis) (Fig. 8.9). The hormonal disturbances of acromegaly and hypothyroidism are acquired and one of the signs may be macroglossia. Amyloid deposition is another condition, usually systemic, in which protein metabolism is disturbed. The amyloid accumulates and infiltrates major organs. Amyloid may occur secondarily in association with malignant tumors. In the tongue

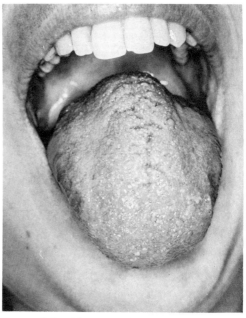

Figure 8.9. Macroglossia associated with angiomatosis of the tongue. The whole tongue was involved with a congenital hemangioma.

Table 8.1.
Macroglossia

Causes (Condition)	Category of Disease
Congenital	
Genetic—mongolism	Developmental
Developmental—hemangioma, lymphangioma	
Idiopathic	
Acquired	
Trauma—inflammatory edema, stomatitis	Inflammatory
Radiation therapy—edema	
Habit—hypertrophy	Hyperplastic
Tumor—neurofibroma	Neoplastic
Hormone disturbance—acromegaly, hypothyroidism (cretinism, myxedema)	Metabolic (systemic)
Metabolic disturbance—amyloid deposits	

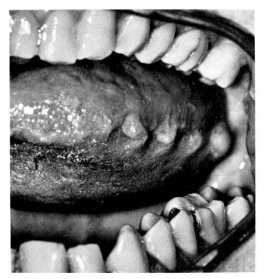

Figure 8.10. Macroglossia and scalloping of lateral border of tongue associated with nervous habit of tongue-thrusting.

it replaces the musculature and causes a macroglossia. Therefore, the dentist may be requested by the patient's physician to biopsy the tongue because it is much more accessible than the other organs that might be involved, to evaluate the possibility of amyloid deposition. The nervous habit of forcing the tongue against the teeth or dentures may result in a hypertrophy of the tissue with enlargement (Fig. 8.10). Many inflammatory situations, particularly in acute stomatitis, yield edema, scalloped tongue and a large, full tongue. Acute herpetic stomatitis and erythema multiforme are examples. Similar edema may result during or following radiation therapy. Finally, there may be gross enlargement with a tumor. In von Recklinghausen's neurofibromatosis, multiple neurofibromas cause a pronounced macroglossia. There are many unknown causes listed as idiopathic. Thus, macroglossia, readily observed, may have many causes. The manifestation of a large tongue may be categorized according to the response of the body into developmental, inflammatory, hyperplastic, neoplastic, or metabolic (systemic) disease. If no observation is made, the pathology will be overlooked.

Bibliography

1. Bhaskar SN: *Synopsis of Oral Pathology*, ed 6. St Louis, Mosby, 1981.
2. Golden A: *Pathology—Understanding Human Disease*. Baltimore, Williams & Wilkins, 1982.
3. Hill RB, LaVia MF: *Principles of Pathobiology*, ed 3. New York, Oxford University Press, 1980.
4. Kerr DA, Ash M: *Oral Pathology: An Introduction to General and Oral Pathology for Hygienists*, ed 4. Philadelphia, Lea & Febiger, 1978.
5. Pindborg JJ: *Pathology of the Dental Hard Tissues*. Philadelphia, Saunders, 1970.
6. Robinson HBG, Miller AS: *Colby, Kerr and Robinson's Color Atlas of Oral Pathology*, ed 4. Philadelphia, Lippincott, 1983.
7. Shafer WG, Hine MK, Levy BM, Tomich CE: *A Textbook of Oral Pathology*, ed 4. Philadelphia, Saunders, 1983.
8. Shklar G, McCarthy P: *Oral Manifestations of Systemic Disease*. Boston, Butterworths, 1976.
9. Walter JB: *An Introduction to the Principles of Disease*. Philadelphia, Saunders, 1977.
10. Wood NK, Goaz PW: *Differential Diagnosis of Oral Lesions*, ed 2. St Louis, Mosby, 1980.
11. Young WG, Sedano HO: *Atlas of Oral Pathology*. Minneapolis, University of Minnesota Press, 1981.

Index

Abrasion, 44
Abscess, 21
  dentoalveolar, 57
  gingival, 58
  palatal, 58
  parulis, 57
  periapical,
    sequelae of pulpitis, 54, 56–58
  periodontal, 57
  pulpal, 54
Accessory teeth, 35–36
Acute herpetic gingivostomatitis, 82–84
Acute necrotizing ulcerative gingivitis, 94–95
Adenomatoid odontogenic tumor, 123
Amalgam tattoo, 130–131
Ameloblastic fibroma, 123
Ameloblastoma, 113, 121–123
Amelogenesis imperfecta, 42–43
Amyloid, 135
Anemias, 132–133
Angiomas, 113, 117
Angular cheilosis, in systemic disease, 132–133
Ankyloglossia, 29
Anodontia, 34
Aphthrous stomatitis, 87–89
Aspirin burn, 90
Atrophic glossitis
  in anemic states, 132
  syphilitic, 96–97, 133
Atrophy, 15–16, 80–81
Attrition, 44

"Bald" tongue, in nutritional deficiencies, 133
Basal cell tumor, 2, 128
Benign and malignant conditions, 111–128
Benign mixed tumor, 120
Bifid tongue, 29
Biopsy, 71–72
Birth defects, 27
Bitewing radiograph, caries, 51
Bulla, 79

Cancer, 17, 111–116
  extraoral, 128
  intraoral, 124, 126–128
  of lip, 125
  oral, 124–128
Candidiasis, 30, 102
Canker sores, 87–89
Carcinogens, 114
Carcinoma, 112–113
  basal cell, 2, 128
  epidermoid or squamous cell, 17, 80, 125–127
Caries, dental, 46–52

Cavernous sinus thrombosis, 63
Cellular structure, 11
Cellulitis, 56–58
Cementoma, 69, 123
Central papillary atrophy, tongue, 29–30
Chancre, primary, syphilis, 96
Cheilosis, angular, in systemic disease, 132–133
Chemical trauma ulcers, 90
Chemotaxis, 19–20
Chickenpox virus, 86
Circulatory disturbance, classification of disease, 12–14
Cleft lip and palate, 27–28
Cleidocranial dysplasia, 34
Clinical examination, 1–10
Cold sores, 83
Collagen formation, following inflammation, 22–23
Concrescence, 37
Condensing osteitis, 64, 124
Congenital malformations, 12, 27
Congenital syphilis, 41, 98
Coxsackie virus, 85
Crust, 81
Cyst(s)
  developmental, 64–68
  gingival, 64–109
  inflammatory, 61–62
  nonodontogenic, 64, 67
  odontogenic, 64–67
  sequelae of pulpitis, 58, 61–62
  traumatic bone, 68
Cyst-like lesions, 68–69
Cytology, oral exfoliative, 72

Degenerative changes, classification of disease, 12–13
Dens in dente, 38
Dental pulp disorders, 52–56
Dentinogenesis imperfecta, 43
Dentoalveolar abscess, sequelae of pulpitis, 56–58
Denture hyperplasia, 93–94
Denture sore mouth, 90, 102
Desquamative gingivitis, 109
Developmental abnormalities, 27–43
Diapedesis, 19–20
Dilaceration, 38–39
Disease classification, 11–12
Dysplasia, epithelial, 103–104, 106, 115

Ectodermal dysplasia, 34
Electrical burns and ulcerations, 89, 91
Emperipolesis, 20–21
Enamel hypoplasia, 39–42
Enamel opacities, 42
Eosinophilic granuloma, 124

Eosinophils, role in inflammation and repair, 22
Epstein's pearls, 109
Epulis, 91
    fissuratum, 93
    giant cell, 92
    granulomatosum, 92
Erosion
    of oral mucosa, 79
    of teeth, 44–45
Erythema multiforme, 110
Erythroblastosis fetalis, 130
Examination
    clinical, 1–10
    extraoral, 1–5
    oral, 5–10
    procedure, 1–2
    technique, 2–10
Exostosis, 33
External resorption, 55
Extraoral cancer, 128
Extraoral examination, 1–5
Exudation, 20–21

Fibroblasts, role in inflammation and repair, 22
Fibroma, 113, 116–117
Fibromatosis gingivae, 32, 116
Fibrosis, following inflammation, 23
Fibrous dysplasia, 123
Fissural cysts, 65, 67
Fissured tongue, 30
Fistula, 57, 59
Fluorosis, 41
Focal sclerosing osteitis, 64, 124
Follicular cysts, 64–65
Fordyce's granules, 5–6, 32, 109
    white lesions associated with, 103, 109
Fungal infections, 102
Furrowed tongue, 30
Fusion of teeth, 37–38

Gangrenous stomatitis, 95
Gemination, 35, 37
Geographic tongue, 30–31
    white lesions associated with, 103, 108
Giant cell epulis, 92
Giant cell granuloma, peripheral, 92
Gingival cyst of newborn, 109
Gingival fibromatosis, hereditary, 32, 116
Gingivitis
    acute necrotizing ulcerative, 94–95
    desquamative, 109
    in systemic disease, 134
Gingivostomatitis, acute herpetic, 82–84
Glands, swollen lymph, 2–5
Glossitis
    atrophic
        in anemia, 132
        syphilitic, 96–97
    median rhomboid, 29, 102
Gonorrhea, 98–99
Granulation tissue, 22–23
Granuloma
    peripheral giant cell, 92
    pyogenic, 91–92
    sequelae of pulpitis, 56, 58
Granulomatous disease, 99–100

Gum boil, 57
Gumma, syphilitic, 96–97

Hairy tongue, 31–32, 103
    white, 103, 108
Hamartoma, 117
Healing, wound, 23–25
Hemangioma, 117
Hematoma, 118
Hereditary gingival fibromatosis, 32, 116
Hereditary neurofibromatosis, multiple, 119
Herpangina, 85–86
Herpes labialis, 83–85
Herpes simplex hominis virus, 81–85
Herpes zoster, 86
Herpetic stomatitis, 82–83
Hyperkeratosis
    in dysplasia, 75, 77, 103
    in leukoplakia, 73–74, 77, 103–105
Hyperplasia, 14
Hyperplastic pulpitis, 54
Hypertrophy, 15
Hypocalcemia, 40
Hypocalcification, 42
Hypoplasia,
    enamel, 39–42
    Turner's, 41

Infectious mononucleosis, 5, 87
Inflammation
    and repair, 19–26
    classification of disease, 11–12
Inflammatory papillary hyperplasia of the palate, 93–94
Internal resorption, 55
Intraoral cancer, 124, 126–128
Iron deficiency anemia, 133
Irritation fibroma, 116–117

Jaws, developmental abnormalities, 33–34

Langhans' giant cells, tuberculosis, 99
Lateral, peg, 41
Leukemia, 134
Leukoedema, white lesions associated with, 108–109
Leukoplakia, 73–74, 78, 103–105
Lichen planus, 77–78, 107–108
Lip
    cancer, 125–126
    double, 28
    pits, 28
Lipoma, 119–120
Ludwig's angina, 63
Lues (syphilis), 95
Lymph nodes, 2–5
Lymphangioma, 113, 119
Lymphocytes, role in inflammation and repair, 20–23

Macrodontia, 35
Macroglossia, 28
    in systemic disease, 134–135
Macrognathia, 33
Macule, 77
Malignant and benign conditions, 111–128
Measles, 86
Median rhomboid glossitis, 29, 102

Melanin pigmentation, normal and malignant, 128–130
Melanoma, 2, 129
Melanotic macule, 130
Mesiodens, 35
Metaplasia, 15–16
Metastasis, 18, 111–112, 115, 128
Microdontia, 35
Microglossia, 29
Micrognathia, 33
Moniliasis, 30, 102
Monocytes, role in inflammation and repair, 21–22
Mucocele, 100–101
Mucosal tag, 5
Mucous membrane pathology, oral, 70–110
Mucous membrane pemphigoid, 110
Mucous patch, syphilis, 96–97
Multiple hereditary neurofibromatosis, 119
Mumps, 87
Mycobacterium tuberculosis, 99–100
Mycotic infections, 102

Neoplasia, 17, 111–116
Neoplasms, classification, 113
Neurofibroma, 119
Neurofibromatosis, multiple hereditary, 119
Neuromas, 119
Neutrophils, role in inflammation and repair, 19–22
Nevus
    melanotic, 129
    white sponge, 32, 108
Nicotinic stomatitis, 105–107
Nodule, 78–79
Noma, 95
Nutritional deficiencies, 132

Odontogenic tumors, 121–123
Odontoma, 121
Opacities, enamel, 42
Oral cancer, 124–128
Oral cavity, benign tumors of, 116–123
Oral cytology, 72–73
Oral examination, 5–10
Oral manifestations of systemic diseases, 132–136
Oral mucosa
    clinical changes, 73, 77–81
    connective tissue changes, 73
    epithelial changes, 73
    microscopic changes, 72–73
    normal, 70–71
Oral mucous membrane pathology, 70–110
Osteitis
    condensing, 64
    focal sclerosing, 64
Osteomyelitis, 62
    Garré's proliferative, 63
Osteoporotic marrow defect, 69

Papillary hyperplasia of the palate, 93–94
Papilloma, 120
Papule, 77–78
Parulis, 57
Pathology, principles of, 11–18
Peg-laterals, 40–41
Pemphigus, 110
Periapical abscess, sequelae of pulpitis, 54, 56–58

Periapical cemental dysplasia, 69, 123
Periapical cyst, sequelae of pulpitis, 58
Periapical granuloma, sequelae of pulpitis, 56, 58
Pericoronitis, 94
Periodontal cysts, 64–67
Peripheral giant cell granuloma, 92
Pernicious anemia, 132–134
Petechiae, 119
Peutz-Jeghers syndrome, 128–129
Pierre-Robin syndrome, 34
Pigmentations, 128–131
Plaque, mucosa, 77
Plasma cells, role in inflammation and repair, 21–22
Pleomorphic adenoma, 120
Polymorphonuclear leukocytes
    role in inflammation and repair, 19–22
Pregnancy tumor, 91
Primary herpetic stomatitis, 82–84
Principles of pathology, 11–18
Pseudocyst, of tonsil, 7
Pulp polyp, 54
Pulp stones, 56
Pulpal irritants, 52
Pulpalgia, 53
Pulpitis, 52–55
    sequelae of, 56–61
Pyogenic granuloma, 91

Radicular cyst, sequelae of pulpitis, 56, 58–62
Ranula, 101
Recurrent aphthous stomatitis, 87–89
Recurrent herpetic infections, 83–85
Restitution, following inflammation, 23

Salivary glands, benign mixed tumor of, 120
Sarcoma, 112–113
Scalloped tongue, 136
Scar, 22–23, 80–81
Scarlet fever stomatitis, 95
Scarring following inflammation, 22–23
Shingles, 86
Sialolith, 101
Sinus, fistulous, 59
Skin, normal, 70
Soft tissue,
    abnormalities, 27–33
    cysts, 64, 67–68
Stevens-Johnson syndrome, 110
Stomatitis
    gangrenous, 95
    migrans, 31
    nicotinic, 105–107
    primary herpetic, 82–84
    Vincent's, 94–95
Supernumerary teeth, 35–36
Syphilis (lues), 95
Systemic diseases, oral manifestations of, 132–136

Teeth
    acquired defects, 43–45
    developmental disturbances, 34–43
    eruption, premature or delayed, 39
    position disturbances, 38–39
    supernumerary, 35–36
Telangiectasias, 119
Tetracycline staining, 129–131

Thermal injury ulcers, 91
Thrush, 102
Tissue growth, 14
Tissue repair, 22–23
Tongue
  "bald," in nutritional deficiencies, 133
  bifid, 29
  fissured or furrowed, 30
  geographic, 30–31
    white lesions associated with, 103, 108
  hairy, 31–32, 103
    white, 103, 108
  scalloped, 136
Tonsils, 6–7
  pseudocysts of, 7
Tooth decay, 46–52
Toothbrush abrasion, 44
Tori, 32–33
Tori mandibularis, 33
Torus palatinus, 33

Traumatic ulcers, 89–91
Trench mouth (acute necrotizing gingivitis), 94–95
Tuberculosis, 99–100
Tumor, 17, 80
  benign, 112–113
  malignant, 112–113
Turner's hypoplasia, 41

Ulceromembranous gingivitis, 94
Ulcers, 26, 73, 78–79, 89–91

Vasodilation, 19–20
Vesicle, 73, 78
Vincent's stomatitis, 94–95
Viral infections of the oral cavity, 81–87
von Recklinghausen's neurofibromatosis, 119

White hairy tongue, 103, 108
White lesions, 102–110
White sponge nevus, 32, 108